For reducing local recurrence
At high risk the cervical cancer

Robot Extended Nerve Sparing Radical Hysterectomy with Extended Pelvic Lymphadenectomy for the Cervical Cancer

Yoon S Lee, Prof.

Kyungpook National University Chilgok Hospital
Gynecologic Cancer Center Daegu, Korea

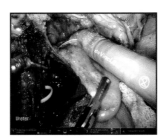
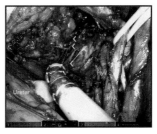

Video Inside!

군자출판사

Robot Extended Nerve Sparing Radical Hysterectomy with Extended Pelvic Lymphadenectomy for the Cervical Cancer

첫 째 판 1쇄 인쇄 | 2018년 1월 3일
첫 째 판 1쇄 발행 | 2018년 1월 11일

지 은 이 이윤순
발 행 인 장주연
출 판 기 획 이성재
편집디자인 김지선
표지디자인 이상희
발 행 처 군자출판사(주)
　　　　　등록 제4-139호(1991. 6. 24)
　　　　　본사 (10881) 파주출판단지 경기도 파주시 회동길 338(서패동 474-1)
　　　　　전화 (031) 943-1888　　팩스 (031) 955-9545
　　　　　홈페이지 | www.koonja.co.kr

ISBN 979-11-5955-267-0

정가 70,000원

Yoon S Lee, Prof.

E mail; yslee@knu.ac.kr

807 Hoguk-ro, Buk-gu,Daegu 41404, Korea

053-200-2114, 053-200-3131 (OPD)

Kyungpook National University Chilgok Hospital

Chief of center for Gynecologic cancer.

Prof. PhD

Gynecologic oncology

Laparoscopic surgery, certified AAGL since late 1990

Robotic surgery since 2008, we used Si and Xi da vinci system

Single port laparoscopic surgery and single port robotic surgery

Vaginal hysterectomy since 1990

Preface

I have performed laparoscopic oncologic surgery since 1994. We published our laparoscopic surgical outcomes at many articles. However, the laparoscopic anatomic structures were still unstable for the education for oncologic surgeons. Fortunately, We performed robot radical hysterectomy since 2008. We expected the robotic radical hysterectomy could reduce the local recurrence of cervical cancer, but our initial long term survival data was similar to the laparoscopic radical hysterectomy. Therefore; we performed the robot assisted total mesometrial resection method, but results were not satisfied than expected. We have changed our method more extensively than previous styles. In this book, I described the conception of rectovaginal ligament, rectal branches of inferior hypogastric plexus with communication with vesical branches, pelvic splanchnic nerves branches and hypogastric branches . It shows many figures for Robot Extended nerve sparing radical hysterectomy with extended pelvic node dissection. I expected that many patients with high risk cervical cancer could be reduced the their local recurrence by our conceptions.

I express my appreciations to my residents, fellows, colleagues, and nurses at OPD and operation rooms. I have performed 700 cases of robotic surgery so far and this book was designed to celebrate.

Yoon S Lee, Prof
2017 Aug 21

Contents

Chapter 1

Chapter 2

Chapter 3

Chapter 4

Chapter 1

Chapter 1

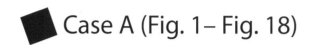 Case A (Fig. 1– Fig. 18)

Conceptions for resection of rectovaginal ligament and preservation of rectal branches of inferior hypogastric plexus.
For purpose of reducing local recurrence of cervical cancer.

BRANCHES OF HYPOGASTRIC ARTERY

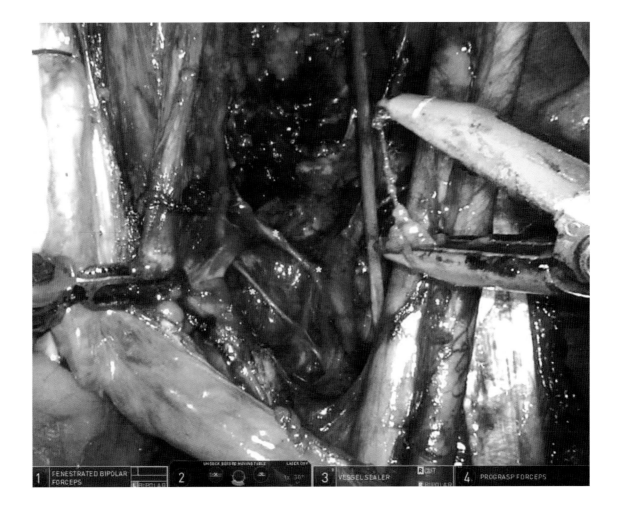

Fig.1

Before traction of hypogastric artery by vessel loop

It is difficult to identify the branches of hypogastric arteries and veins. It is necessary to cut braches of branches of vein (*)

Chapter 1

BRANCHES OF HYPOGASTRIC ARTERY

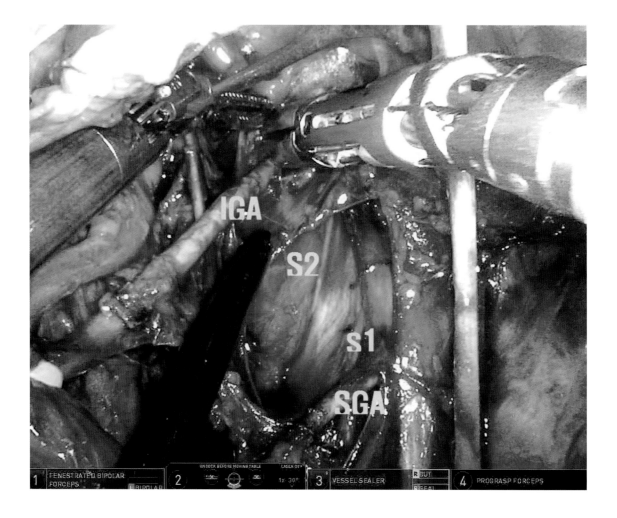

Fig. 2

After traction of hypogastric artery by vessel loop

1. superior gluteal artery-originate between lumbosacral trunk and sacral nerve 1st.
2. common trunk of inferior gluteal artery and internal pudendal artery-originate between sacral nerve 2nd and 3rd (see Fig. 79)
3. identify accompanying veins

BRANCHES OF HYPOGASTRIC ARTERY

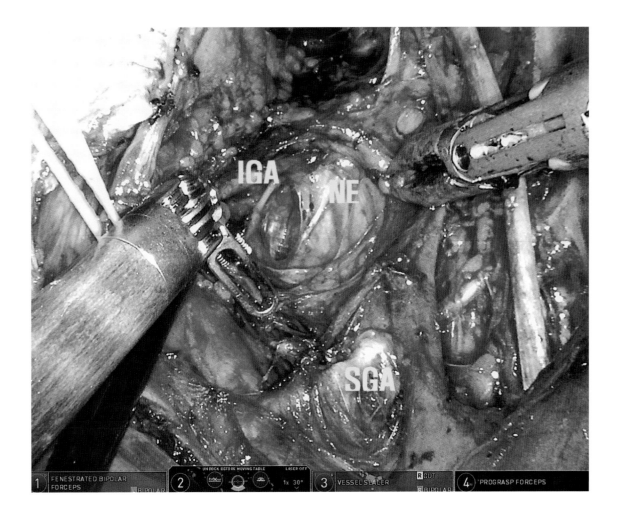

Fig. 3

After traction of hypogastric artery by vessel loop

1. superior gluteal artery-originate between lumbosacral trunk and sacral nerve 1st.
2. common trunk of inferior gluteal artery and internal pudendal artery-originate between sacral nerve 2nd and 3rd (see Fig. 79)
3. pelvic splanchnic nerves=Nervi erigentes from sacral nerve 2nd(NE)
   Tip of vessel sealer indicated branches of hypogastric vein

Chapter 1

BRANCHES OF HYPOGASTRIC ARTERY

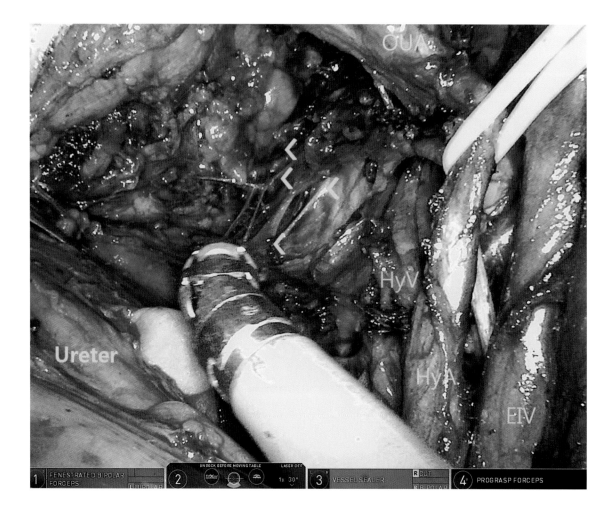

Fig. 4

After traction of right hypogastric artery by vessel loop

Several branches of pelvic splanchnic nerves(<) between paravesical and pararectal space, And hypogastric artery was retracted with yellow loop

- PSN(pelvic splanchnic nerves)
- HyA(hypogastric artery)
- HyV(hypogastric vein)
- EIA(external iliac artery)
- EIV(external iliac vein)
- O(obturator nerve)
- OUA(obliterate umbilical artery)

ISOLATION OF HN FROM IHP, RIGHT

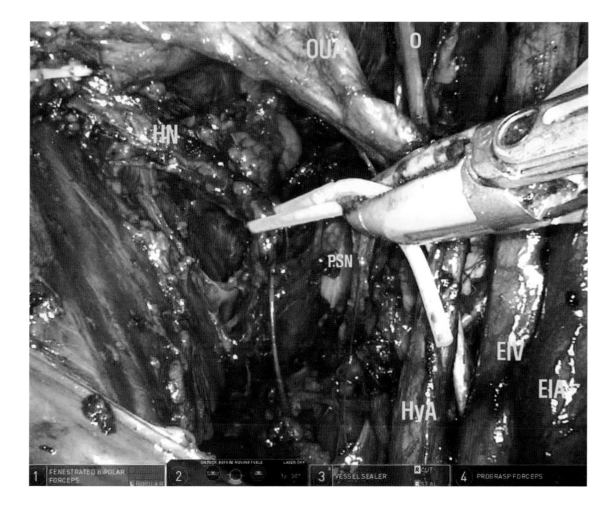

Fig. 4-1

After traction of right hypogastric artery by vessel loop

Isolation of Hypogastric nerve from inferior hypogastric plexus (short yellow vessel loop)

See the communicated between the PSN and NH from IHP

- PSN(pelvic splanchnic nerves)
- HyA(hypogastric artery
- EIA(external iliac artery)
- EIV(external iliac vein)
- O(obturator nerve)
- OUA(obliterate umbilical artery)

Chapter 1

ISOLATION OF HN FROM IHP, RIGHT

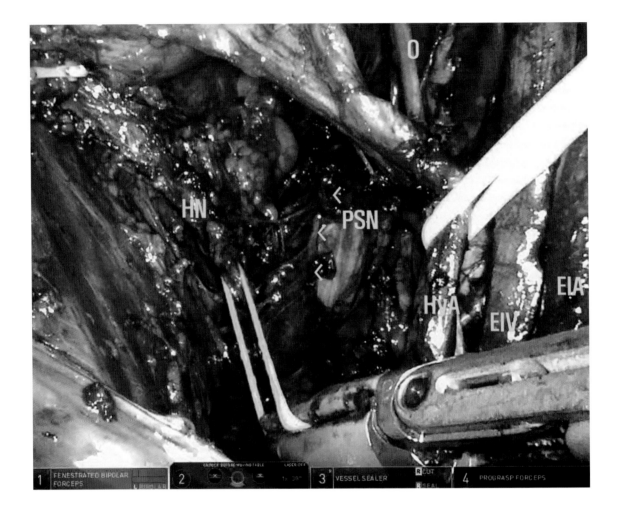

Fig. 4-2

After traction of hypogastric artery by vessel loop

Isolation of right Hypogastric nerve and inferior hypogastric plexus (yellow vessel loop)

See the communicated between the PSN and NH from IHP

- PSN(pelvic splanchnic nerves)
- HyA(hypogastric artery
- EIA(external iliac artery)
- EIV(external iliac vein)
- O(obturator nerve)

BRANCHES OF HYPOGASTRIC ARTERY, LEFT

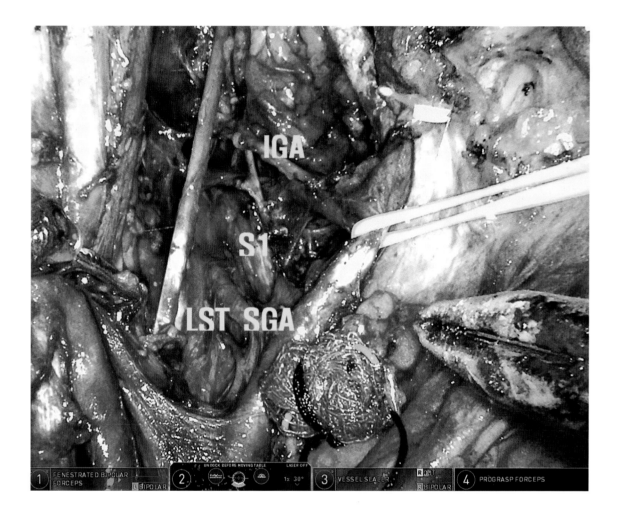

Fig. 5

After traction of hypogastric artery by vessel loop (eft side)

1. superior gluteal artery-originate between lumbosacral trunk (LST) and sacral nerve 1st.(S1)
2. common trunk of inferior gluteal artery and internal pudendal artery-originate between sacral nerve 2nd and 3rd

Chapter 1

HYPOGASTRIC NERVE, IHP, LEFT

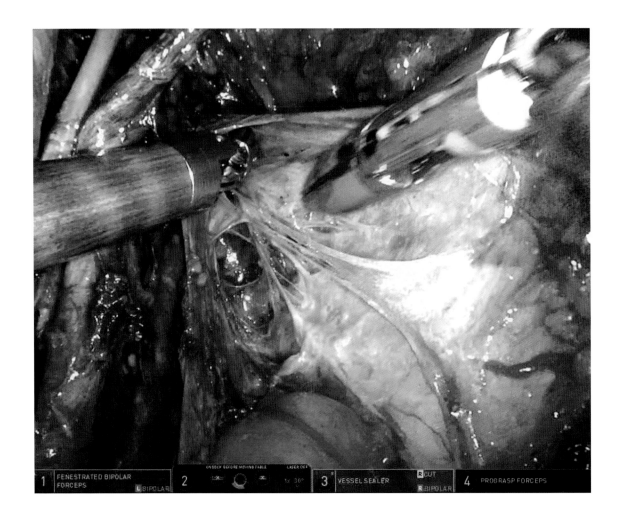

Fig. 5-1

Isolation of left hypogastric nerve from inferior hypogastric plexus

HYPOGASTRIC NERVE, IHP, LEFT

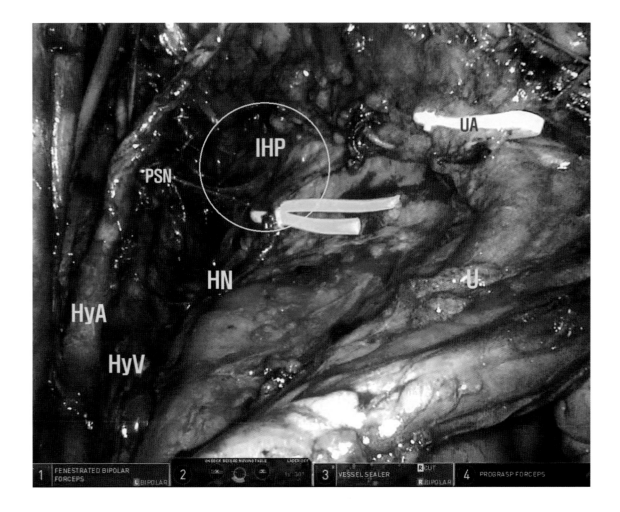

Fig. 5-2

Isolation of left hypogastric nerve and inferior hypogastric plexus (yellow vessel loop)

Identify the communication between the pelvic splanchnic nerves (PSN) and IHP

- HyA(hypogastric artery)
- HyV(hypogastric vein)
- UA(cur end of uterine artery)
- U(ureter)

Chapter 1

RECTOVAGINAL LIGAMENT, RIGHT

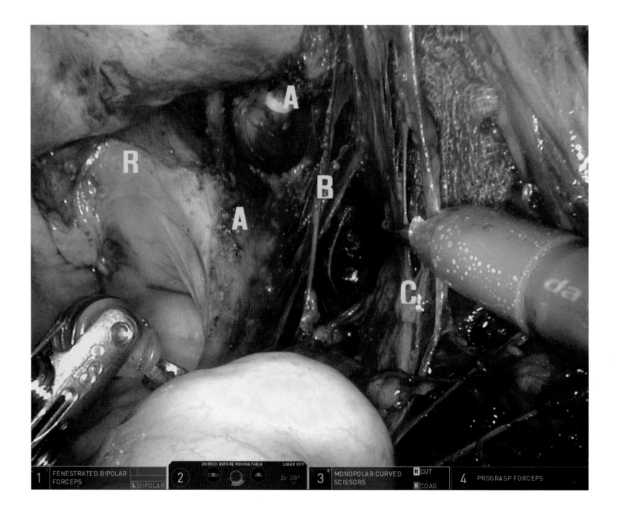

Fig. 6

After resection of of the Rectovaginal ligament

- A (resected vaginal and rectal end of rectovaginal ligament)
- B (rectal branches of inferior hypogastric plexus)
- C (hypogastric nerve and inferior hypogastric plexus)
- R (rectum)

RECTOVAGINAL LIGAMENT, RIGHT

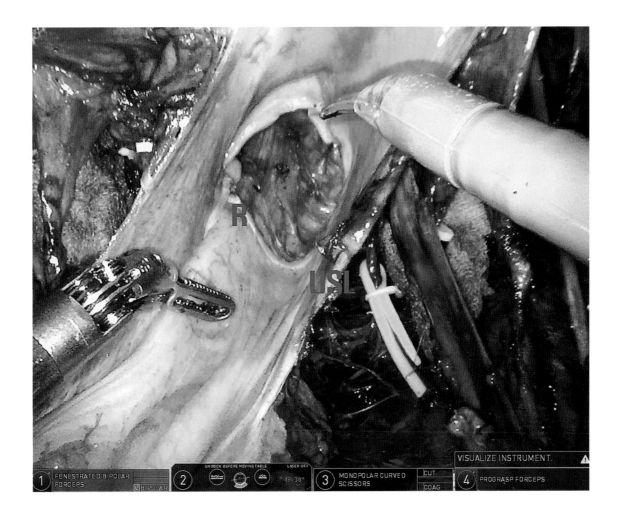

Fig. 7

After dissection of rectovaginal space, identify the rectum and pararectal space and medial border of rectovaginal ligament and uterosacral ligament. Yellow vessel loop indicated Hypogastric nerve and IHP

• U S L(uterosacral ligament)

Chapter 1

RECTOVAGINAL LIGAMENT, RIGHT

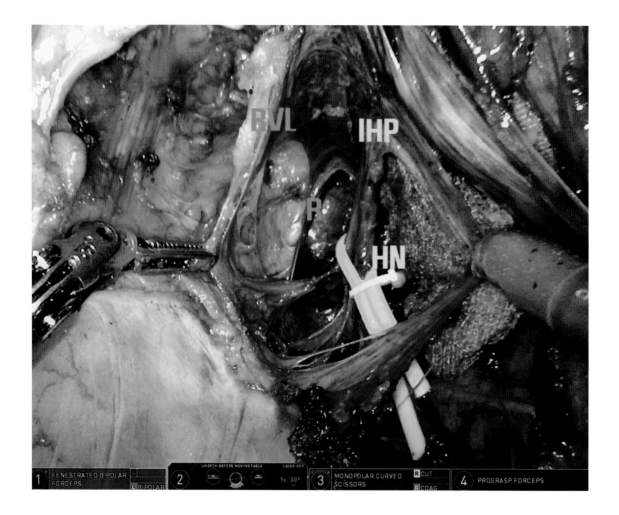

Fig. 8

After cutting the uterosacral ligament, we can identify medial and lateral margin of rectovaginal ligament(RVL), rectal branches(R) of inferior hypogastric plexus(IHP) and hypogastric nerve(HN) from inferior hypogastric plexus. Rectal branches of IHP was separated from lateral margin of RVL by sharp scissors dissection. This procedures continue to the pelvic floor, levator ani muscle.

Superficial branches of hypogastric nerve from Superior hypogastric plexus.was retracted with Tip of scissors.

Tip of bipolar forceps indicated the resection line of RVL.

RECTOVAGINAL LIGAMENT, RIGHT

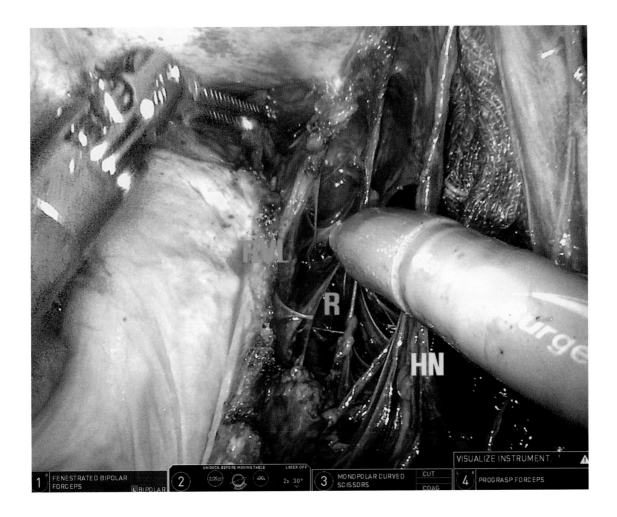

Fig. 8-1

Another cases who did not mark with vessel loop

After cutting the uterosacral ligament, we can identify medial and lateral margin of rectovaginal ligament, rectal branches of inferior hypogastric plexus (R) and hypogastric nerve from inferior hypogastric plexus (HN)

• RVL(rectovaginal ligament)

Chapter 1

RECTOVAGINAL LIGAMENT, RIGHT

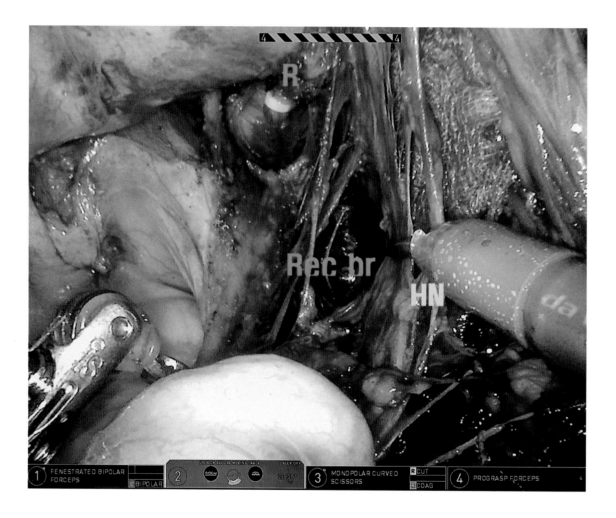

Fig. 8-2

Another cases who did not mark with vessel loop

After cutting the medial and lateral margin of rectovaginal ligament, we can identify rectal branches of inferior hypogastric plexus (Recbr) and hypogastric nerve(HN) from inferior hypogastric plexus (IHP)R (resected end at vaginal part of rectovaginal ligament, Hemo-lok)

RECTOVAGINAL LIGAMENT, RIGHT

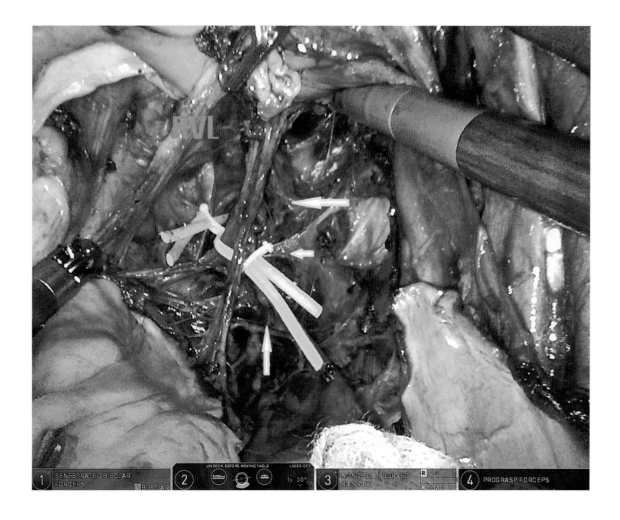

Fig. 9

After cutting the uterosacral ligament, we can identify medial and lateral margin of rectovaginal ligament, rectal branches of inferior hypogastric plexus(blue vessel loop) and hypogastric nerve from inferior hypogastric plexus(yellow vessel loop), branches of pelvic splanchnic nerves(yellow arrow) which were communicated with each other.

Chapter 1

RECTOVAGINAL LIGAMENT, RIGHT

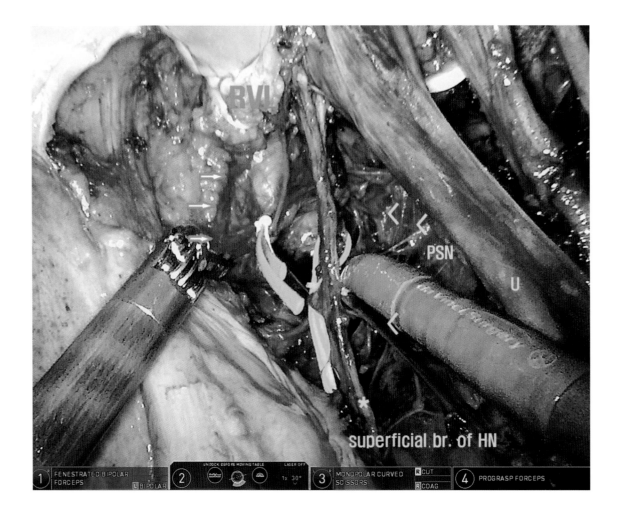

Fig. 10

After cutting the rectovaginal ligament, we can identify cut end of rectovaginal ligament, rectal part(green arrow) and vaginal part(RVL). rectal branches of inferior hypogastric plexus(blue vessel loop) and hypogastric nerve from inferior hypogastric plexus(yellow vessel loop), branches of pelvic splanchnic nerves(PSN)

Rectal branches and HN from IHP were isolated from pelvic floor.

* indicated superficial branches of HN

• U(ureter)

RECTOVAGINAL LIGAMENT, RIGHT

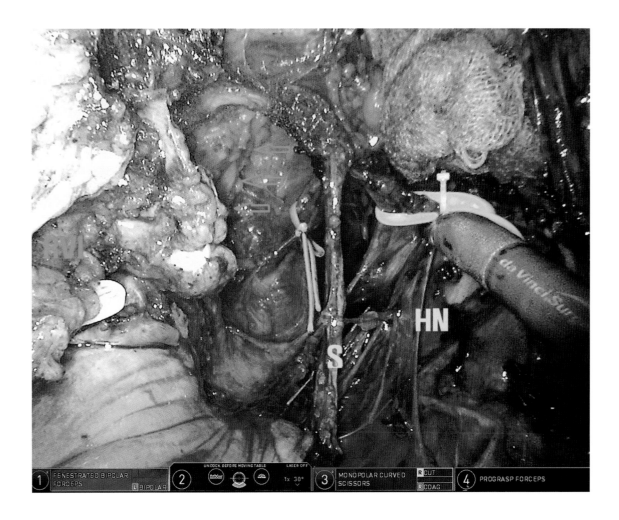

Fig. 11

After dividing anterior and posterior vesicouterine ligament, we can identify cut end of rectovaginal ligament, rectal part (green arrow) and vaginal part(RVL). rectal branches of inferior hypogastric plexus (blue vessel loop) and hypogastric nerve from inferior hypogastric plexus (yellow vessel loop), superficial branches of hypogastric nerve(S), branches of pelvic splanchnic nerves.(not visible)

Chapter 1

RECTOVAGINAL LIGAMENT, LEFT

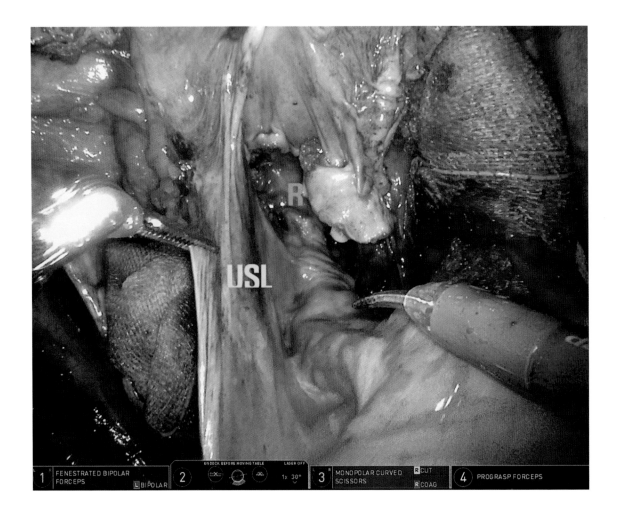

Fig. 12

Resection of Left side of rectovaginal ligament was followed by superficial resection of uterosacral ligament.

RECTOVAGINAL LIGAMENT, LEFT

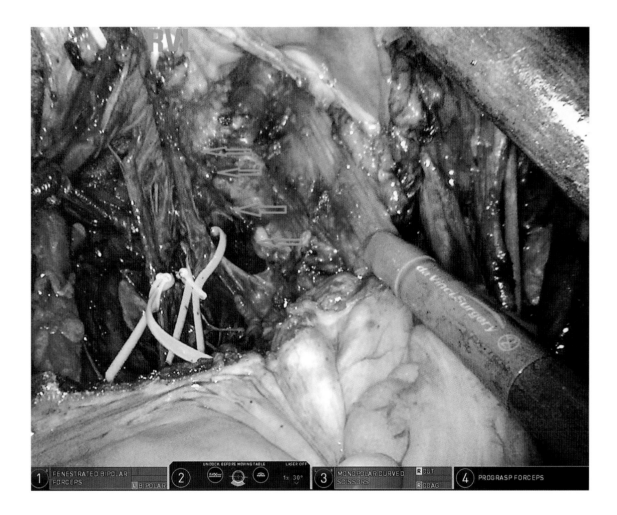

Fig. 13

Resection of Left side of rectovaginal ligament

After cutting the rectovaginal ligament, we can identify cut end of rectovaginal ligament, rectal part (green arrow) and vaginal part(RVL), rectal branches of inferior hypogastric plexus(blue vessel loop) and hypogastric nerve from inferior hypogastric plexus (yellow vessel loop), branches of pelvic splanchnic nerves (not visible)

Chapter 1

RECTOVAGINAL LIGAMENT, LEFT

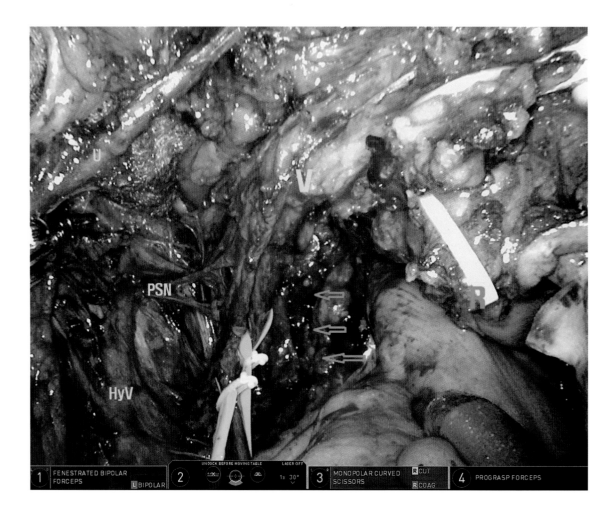

Fig. 14

Resection of Left side of rectovaginal ligament

After dividing anterior and posterior vesicouterine ligament, we can identify cut end of rectovaginal ligament, rectal part(green arrow) and vaginal part(R, Hemo-lok). rectal branches of inferior hypogastric plexus(blue vessel loop) and hypogastric nerve from inferior hypogastric plexus(yellow vessel loop), branches of pelvic splanchnic nerves(PSN), vesical branches of inferior hypogastric plexus(V)
HyV(hypogastric vein)

RECTOVAGINAL LIGAMENT, RIGHT

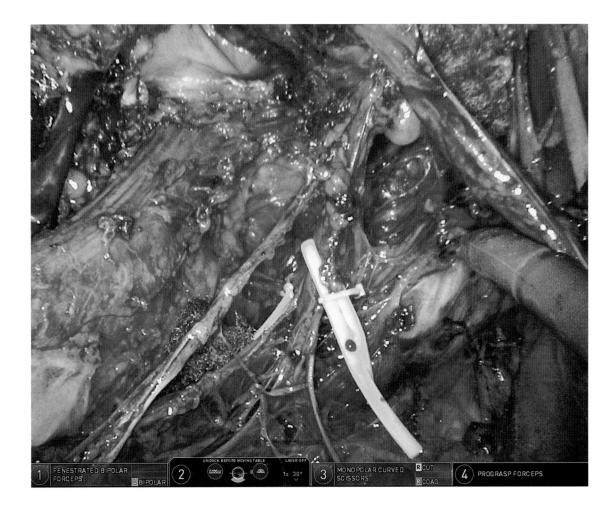

Fig. 15

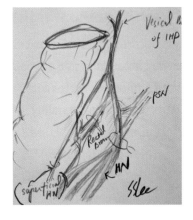

After removal of uterus, final operative view-right side

Communication with rectal branches of inferior hypogastric plexus(blue vessel loop), hypogastric nerve from inferior hypogastric plexus(yellow vessel loop),vesical branches of IHP and branches of pelvic splanchnic nerves

Diagram 1

Chapter 1

RECTOVAGINAL LIGAMENT, RIGHT

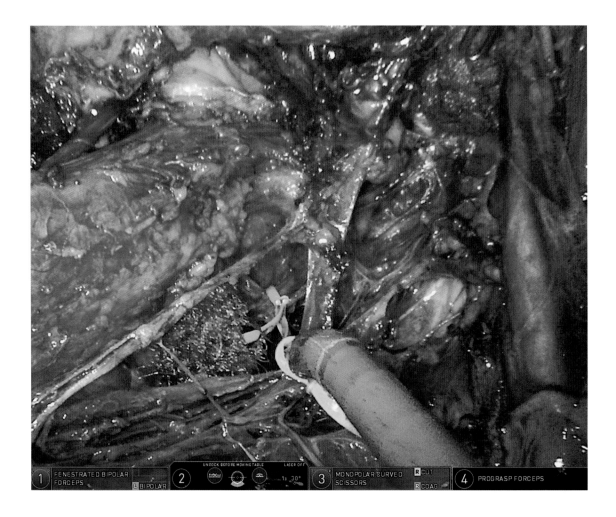

Fig. 16

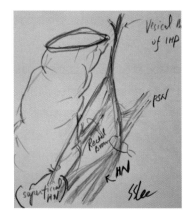

After removal of uterus, final operative view-right side

Communication with rectal branches of inferior hypogastric plexus(blue vessel loop), hypogastric nerve from inferior hypogastric plexus(yellow vessel loop), vesical branches of IHP and branches of pelvic splanchnic nerves

Diagram 1

RECTOVAGINAL LIGAMENT, RIGHT

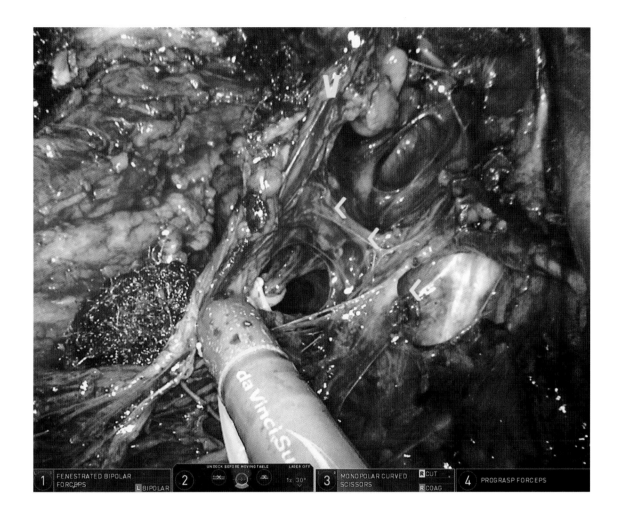

Fig. 17

After removal of uterus, final operative view-right side

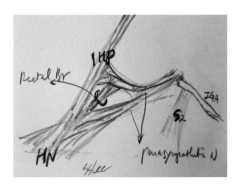

Communication with rectal branches of inferior hypogastric plexus(blue vessel loop), hypogastric nerve from inferior hypogastric plexus(yellow vessel loop), vesical branches of IHP(V) and branches of pelvic splanchnic nerves (<)

Diagram 2

Chapter 1

RECTOVAGINAL LIGAMENT, RIGHT

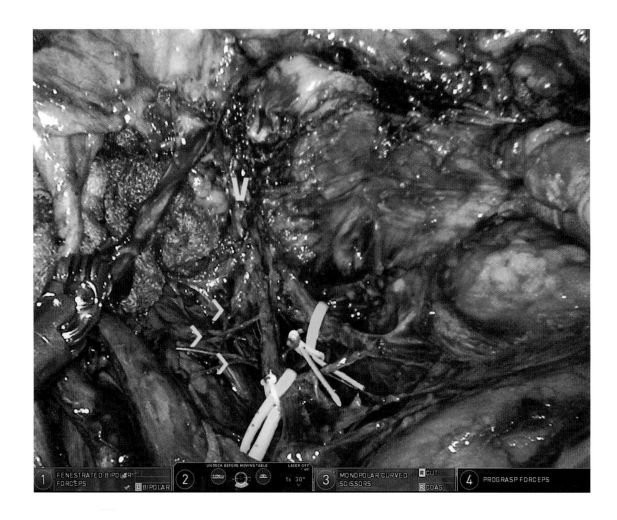

Fig. 18

After removal of uterus, final operative view–left side

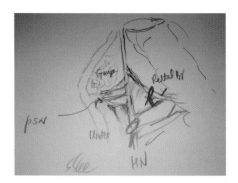

Communication with rectal branches of inferior hypogastric plexus(blue vessel loop), hypogastric nerve from inferior hypogastric plexus (yellow vessel loop), vesical branches of IHP(V) and branches of pelvic splanchnic nerves (>)

Diagram 3

■ Case B (Fig. 19 – Fig. 63)

**Conception of resection of rectovaginal
ligament and preservation of rectal
branches of inferior hypogastric plexus
Preservation of superior hypogastric plexus
Inframesenteric paraaortic node dissection
Extended pelvic node dissection
Vesicouterine ligament dissection
Paravaginal dissection
For purpose of reducing local recurrence in
the cervical cancer**

Chapter 1

INFRAMESENTERIC PARAAORTIC NODE DISSECTION

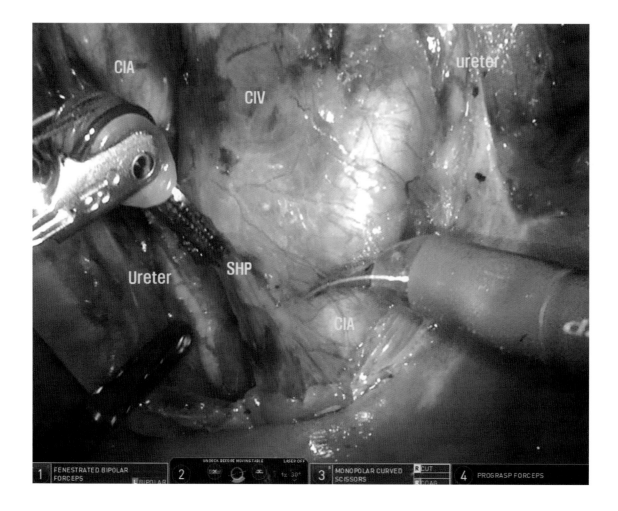

Fig. 19

Preservation of superior hypogastric plexus (SHP) at subaortic area.

After lateral traction of sigmoid mesentery to left side, we identify the SHP. SHP was elevated with Bipolar forceps.

- CIA(common iliac artery)
- CIV(common iliac vein)
- P(promontory)

INFRAMESENTERIC PARAAORTIC NODE DISSECTION

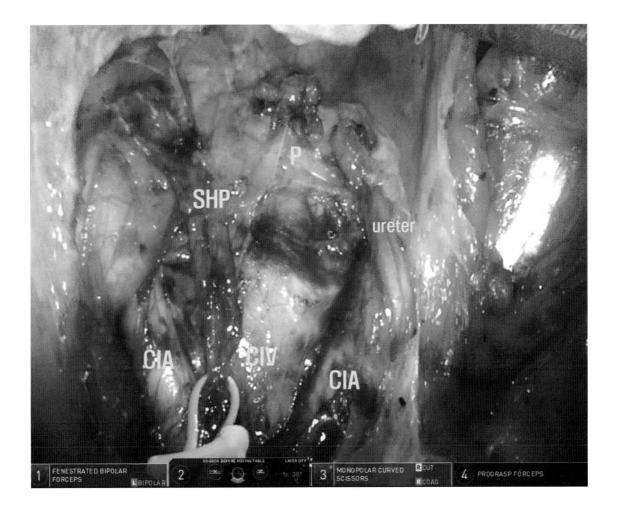

Fig. 20

Preservation and isolation of superior hypogastric plexus(SHP) (long yellow vessel loop)

- CIA(common iliac artery)
- CIV(common iliac vein)
- P(promontory)

Chapter 1

INFRAMESENTERIC PARAAORTIC NODE DISSECTION

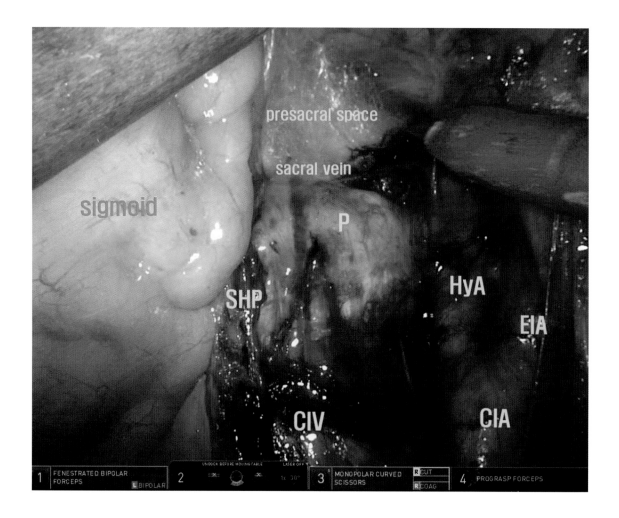

Fig. 21

Preservation of superior hypogastric plexus (yellow vessel loop)

Dissected the right part of presacral nodes around promontory, right common(CIA) and medial part of hypogastric artery(HyA).

• CIA(common iliac artery)

• CIV(common iliac vein)

• P(promontory)

INFRAMESENTERIC PARAAORTIC NODE DISSECTION

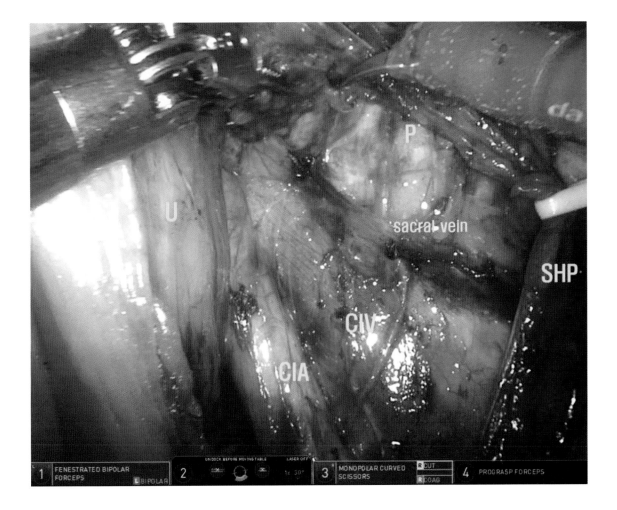

Fig. 22

Preservation of superior hypogastric plexus(SHP) (yellow vessel loop)

Dissected the nodes around left part of presacral nodes at promontory, left common iliac vein and artery (CIV, CIA)

- CIA(common iliac artery)
- CIV(common iliac vein)
- P(promontory)

Chapter 1

INFRAMESENTERIC PARAAORTIC NODE DISSECTION

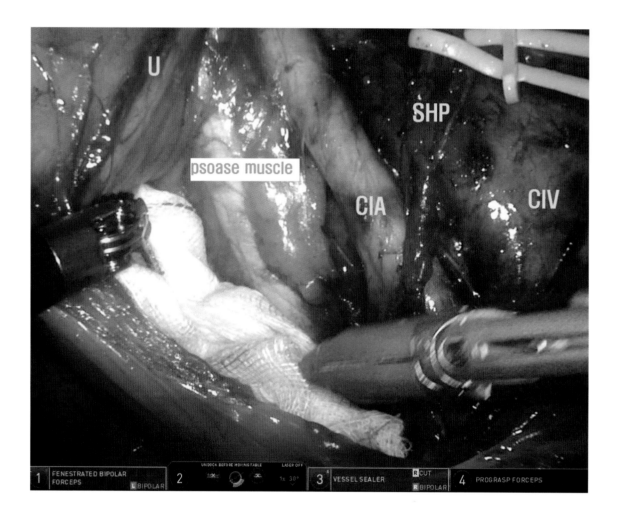

Fig. 23

Preservation of superior hypogastric plexus (yellow vessel loop)

After retraction of left ureter by gauze, we removed the nodes at left common, inframesenteric nodes

- CIA(common iliac artery)
- CIV(common iliac vein)
- P(promontory)

INFRAMESENTERIC PARAAORTIC NODE DISSECTION

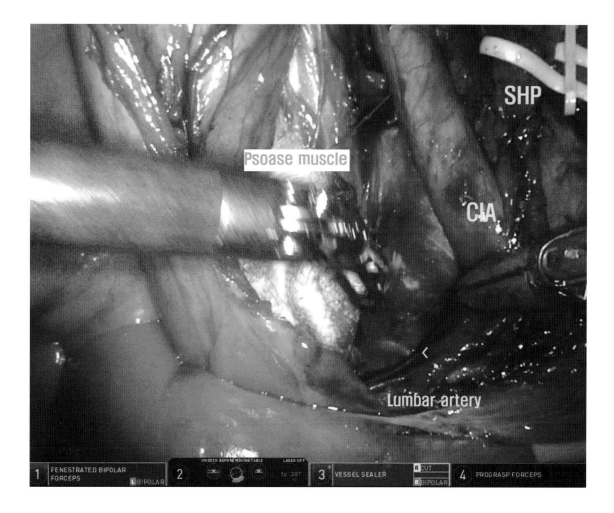

Fig. 24

Preservation of superior hypogastric plexus (yellow vessel loop)

After retraction of left ureter by gauze, nodes were removed at left common, inframesenteric nodes. There were lumbar artery after retraction of CIA by Vessel sealer.

- CIA(common iliac artery)
- CIV(common iliac vein)
- P(promontory)

Chapter 1

INFRAMESENTERIC PARAAORTIC NODE DISSECTION

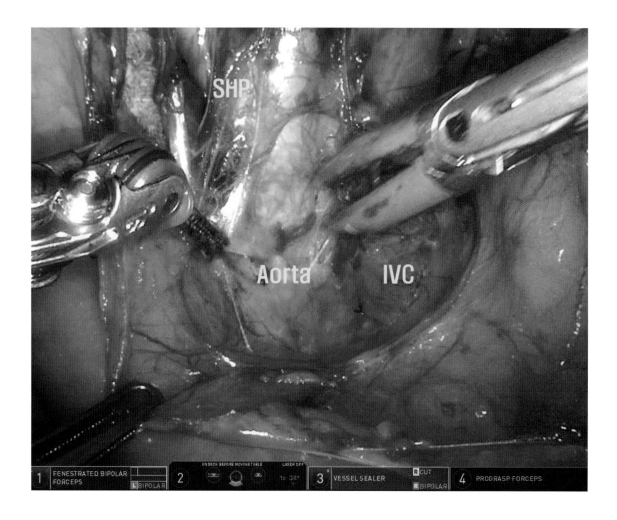

Fig. 25

Preservation of superior hypogastric plexus(yellow vessel loop)

Removed the nodes at paraaortic and right common iliac nodes

INFRAMESENTERIC PARAAORTIC NODE DISSECTION

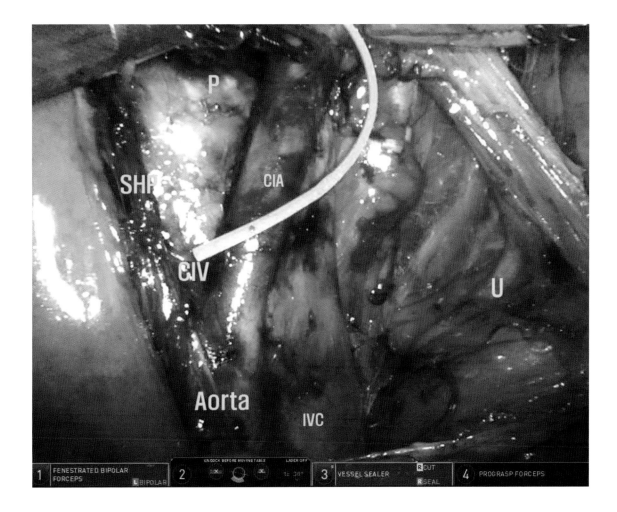

Fig. 26

Preservation of superior hypogastric plexus (yellow vessel loop)

Removed the nodes at paraaortic and right common iliac nodes. This Fig.ure showed after lower paraaortic node dissection.

• CIA(common iliac artery)

• CIV(common iliac vein)

• P(promontory)

• U(ureter)

Chapter 1

RIGHT EXTENDED PELVIC NODE DISSECTION

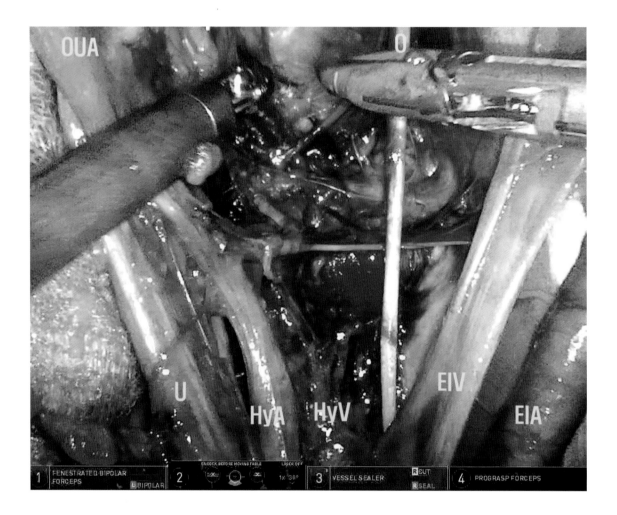

Fig. 27

To dissect more extensively, we used vessel sealer instrument and divided the vessel without excessive bleeding.

We removed the nodes by pulling and traction of the nodal tissues with tip of bipolar or vessel sealer.

• HyA(hypogastric artery)

• HyV(hypogastric vein)

• EIA(external iliac artery)

• EIV(external iliac vein)

• O(obturator nerve)

RIGHT EXTENDED PELVIC NODE DISSECTION

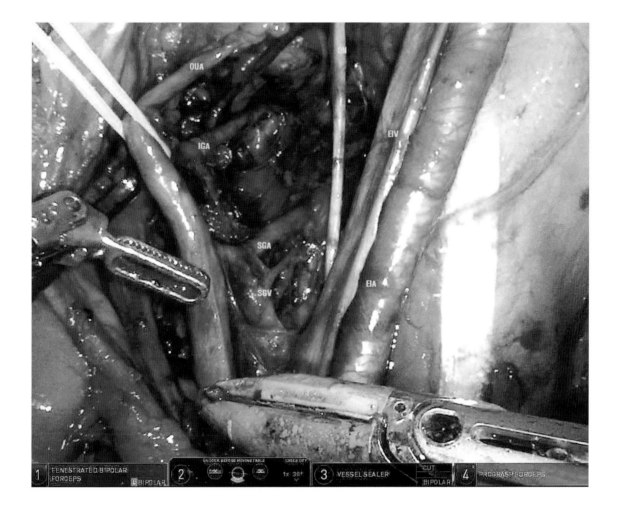

Fig. 28

To dissect more extensively, we used vessel loop which retracted the hypogastric artery by 3rd robotic arm, then branches of hypogastric arteries and veins were identified more clearly.

- IGA(inferior gluteal artery)
- SGA(superior gluteal artery)
- SGV(superior gluteal vein)
- OUA(obliterated umbilical artery)

- ON (obtrurator nerve)
- EIA (external iliac artery)
- EIV(external iliac vein)

Chapter 1

RIGHT EXTENDED PELVIC NODE DISSECTION

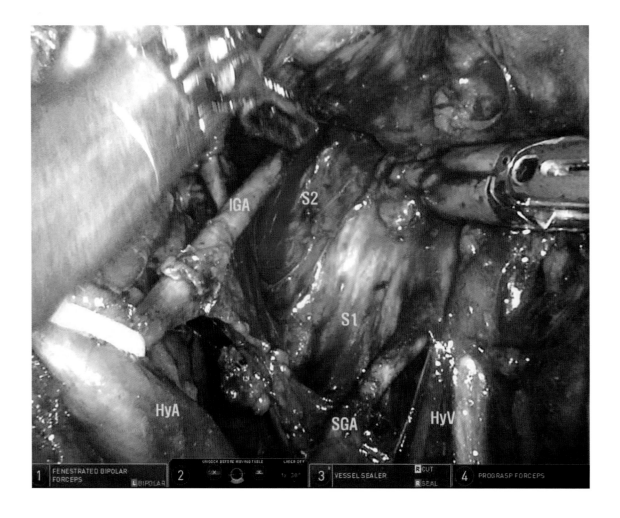

Fig. 29

To dissect more extensively, we used vessel loop which retracted the hypogastric artery by 3rd robotic arm, then branches of hypogastric arteries, veins and sacral nerves were identified more clearly. SGA was supplied to superior gluteal muscles between S1 and LST. Common trunk of IGA and Internal pudendal artery was inserted between S2 and S3.

- IGA(inferior gluteal artery)
- SGA(superior gluteal artery)
- S1(sacral nerve 1st)
- S2(sacral nerve 2nd)
- LST(lumbosacral trunk)

- HyA(hypogastric artery)
- HyV(hypogastric vein)
- EIA(external iliac artery)
- EIV(external iliac vein)

RIGHT EXTENDED PELVIC NODE DISSECTION

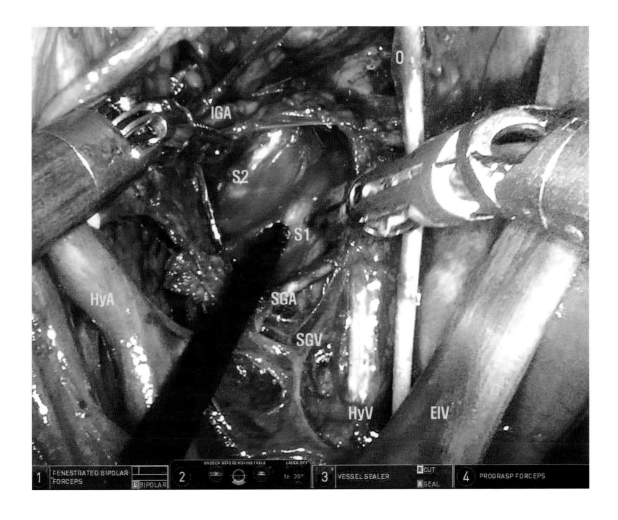

Fig. 30

To dissect more extensively, we used vessel loop which retracted the hypogastric artery by 3rd robotic arm, then branches of hypogastric arteries, veins and sacral nerves were identified more clearly. After removal of thin fascia over Sacral nerve, It was easy to identify the Sacral nerve 2nd (S2)

- IGA(inferior gluteal artery)
- SGA(superior gluteal artery)
- SGV(superior gluteal vein)
- S1(sacral nerve 1st)
- S2(sacral nerve 2nd)

- HyA(hypogastric artery)
- HyV(hypogastric vein)
- EIA(external iliac artery)
- EIV(external iliac vein)

Chapter 1

CARDINAL LIGAMENT DISSECTION, RIGHT

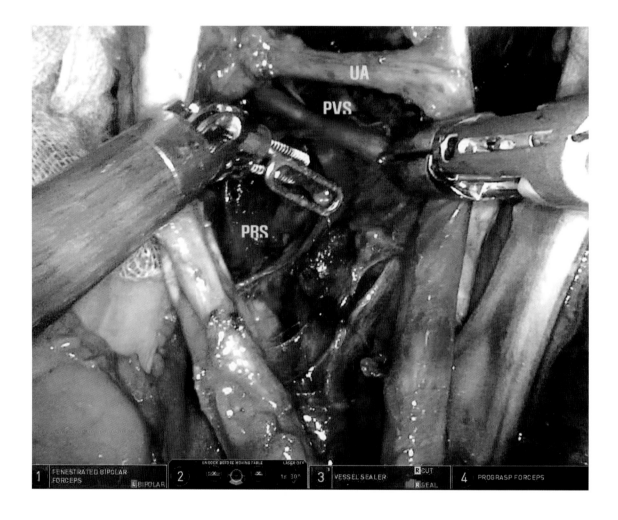

Fig. 31

Cardinal ligament which contained uterine artery(UA) and several branches of veins to the hypogastric vein was situated between the paravesical space(PVS) and pararectal space(PRS)

CARDINAL LIGAMENT DISSECTION
RIGHT EXTENDED PELVIC NODE DISSECTION

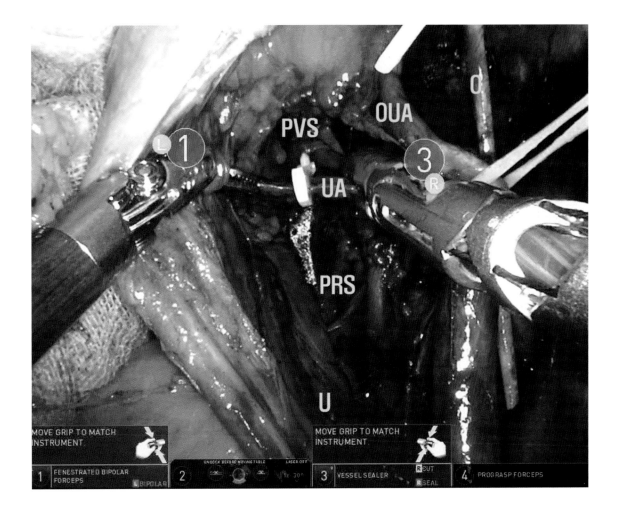

Fig. 32

Uterine artery was divided by vessel sealer and distal part of Uterine artery was marked by hemo lok

• OUA(obliterated umbilical artery)

• O(obtrurator nerve)

• U(ureter)

Chapter 1

CARDINAL LIGAMENT DISSECTION
RIGHT EXTENDED PELVIC NODE DISSECTION

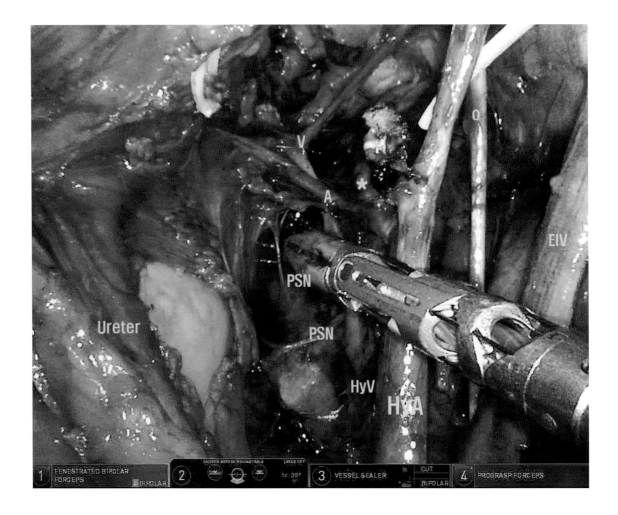

Fig. 33

Cardinal ligament which contained uterine artery (UA) and several branches tohypogastric vein was situated between the paravesical space (PVS) and pararectal space (PRS). In this case, there was one artery and one vein were located in the cardinal ligament, it was rare anatomic variation.

PSN (pelvic splanchnic nerves) were located below the vessel.

* indicated anterior branches of Hypogastric artery.

- HyA (hypogastric artery)
- HyV(hypogastric vein)
- EIA(external iliac artery)

- EIV(external iliac vein)
- O(obturator nerve)
- Hemo lok(cut end of uterine artery)

CARDINAL LIGAMENT DISSECTION
RIGHT EXTENDED PELVIC NODE DISSECTION

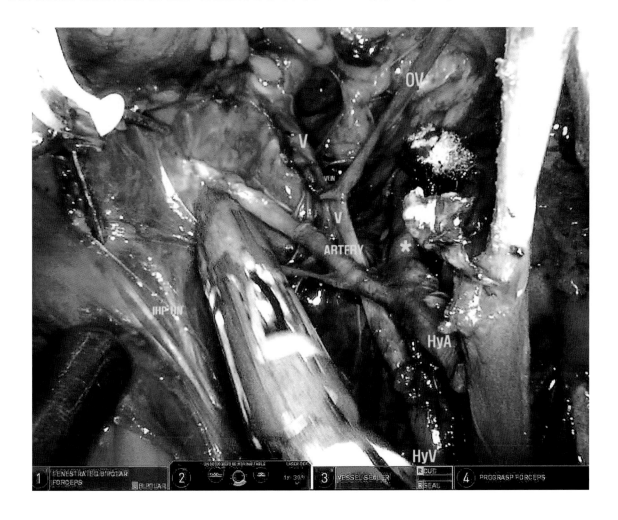

Fig. 34

Cardinal ligament which contained uterine artery (UA) and several branches of veins to the hypogastric vein was situated between the paravesical space (PVS) and pararectal space (PRS)

In this case, there was one artery and one vein were located in the cardinal ligament, it was rare anatomic variation.

* indicated anterior branches of Hypogastric artery.(common trunk of inferior gluteal and internal pudendal artery)

- HyA(hypogastric artery)
- HyV(hypogastric vein)
- EIA(external iliac artery)

- EIV(external iliac vein)
- O(obturator nerve)

Chapter 1

HN FROM IHP, RIGHT

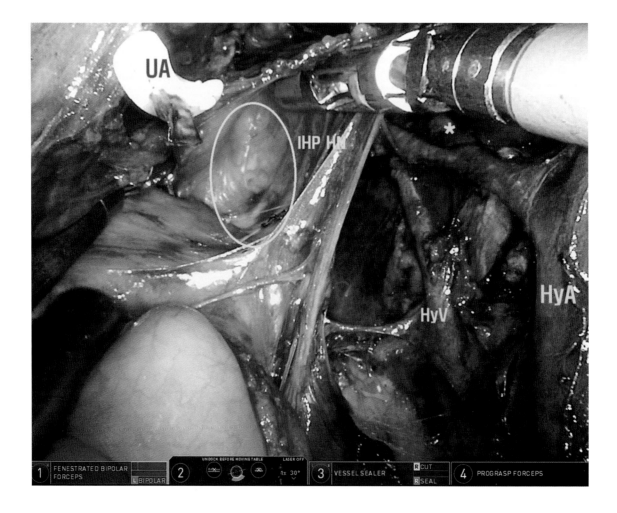

Fig. 35

Hypogastric nerve from IHP (Neural plane) were separated from mesoureter plane to the pelvic floor. Round circle area was Okabayashi space.
Round circle indicated pelvic floor muscle.

- HyA(hypogastric artery)
- HyV(hypogastric vein),
- * indicated anterior branches of Hypogastric artery.
- UA(uterine artery)

HN FROM IHP, RIGHT

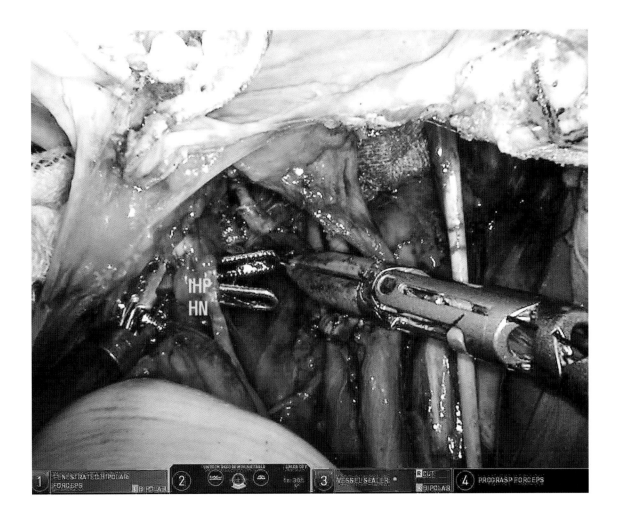

Fig. 36

Hypogastric nerve from IHP were isolated from mesoureter plane to the pelvic floor muscle. These nerves were isolated above pelvic floor muscle. This neural plane was rather thick and firm to perforate. In these thick, firm neural plane protected the local lateral spread of cancer.

Chapter 1

HN FROM IHP, RIGHT

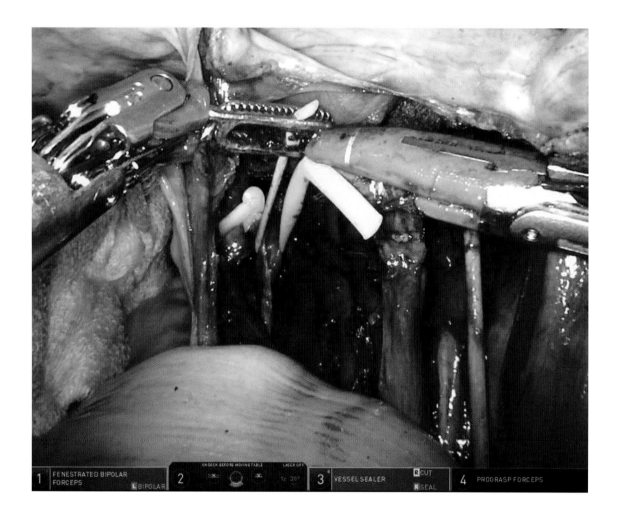

Fig. 37

Neural plane (hypogastric nerve from IHP) were isolated from mesoureter plane to the pelvic floor muscle(yellow vessel loop), then elevated.

RECTOVAGINAL LIGAMENT DISSECTION, RIGHT
RIGHT EXTENDED PELVIC NODE DISSECTION

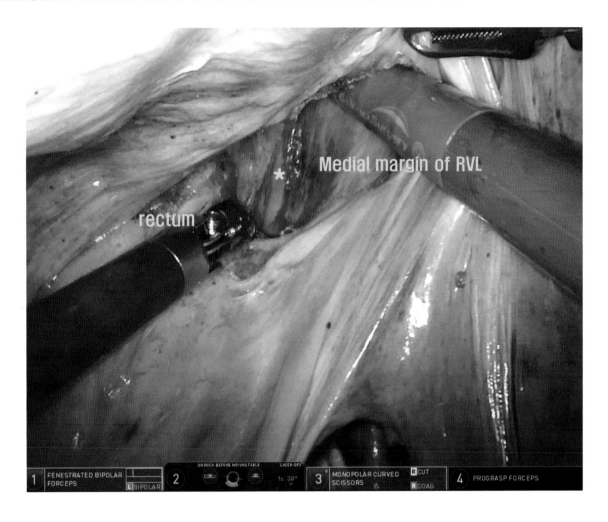

Fig. 38

After dissecting rectovaginal space, identified the medial margin of rectovaginal ligament(RVL)

* indicated muscle of pelvic floor lateral to rectum

Chapter 1

RECTOVAGINAL LIGAMENT DISSECTION, RIGHT
RIGHT EXTENDED PELVIC NODE DISSECTION

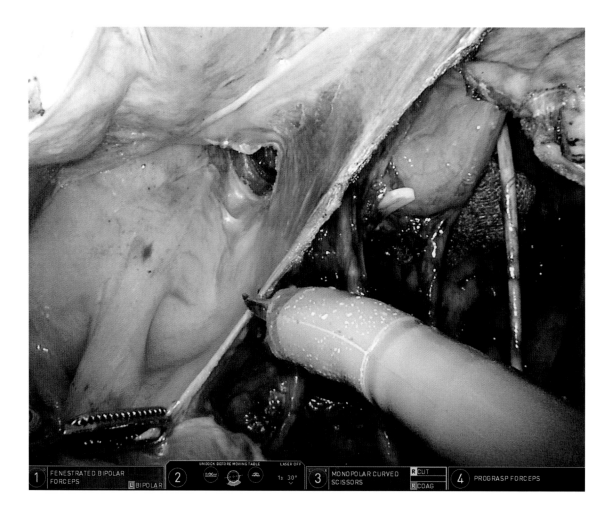

Fig. 39

After dissection of rectovaginal space, identify the rectum and pararectal space and medial border of rectovaginal ligament and uterosacral ligament. then cut uterosacral ligament and identify the rectovaginal ligament .

RECTOVAGINAL LIGAMENT DISSECTION, RIGHT
RIGHT EXTENDED PELVIC NODE DISSECTION

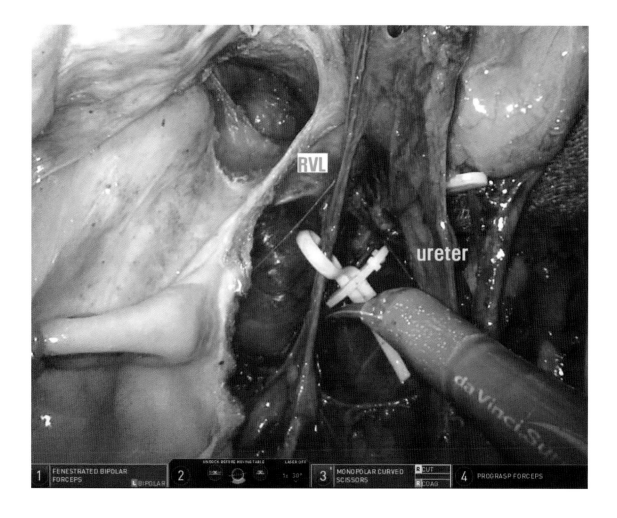

Fig. 40

After dissecting uterosacral ligament and identify the rectovaginal ligament (RVL) which located deeper than the HN from IHP (yellow vessel loop)

Rectal branches of IHP was located at lateral margin RLV.

Yellow vessel loop indicated Hypogastric nerve from IHP

Chapter 1

RECTOVAGINAL LIGAMENT DISSECTION, RIGHT
RIGHT EXTENDED PELVIC NODE DISSECTION

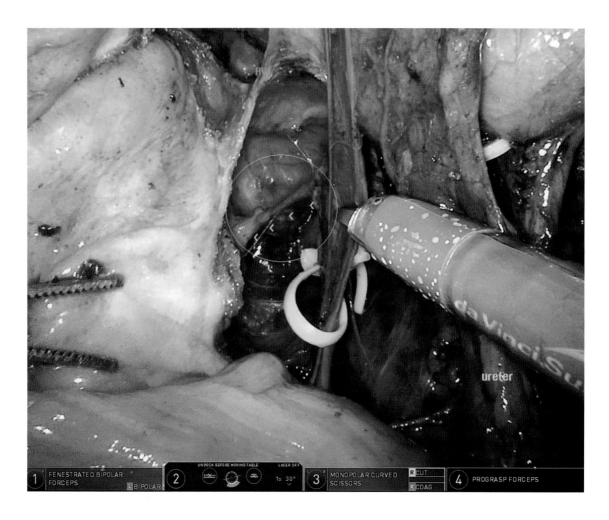

Fig. 41

From the lateral margin of Rectovaginal ligament(RVL) we can identify and separate the rectal branches of IHP(round circle) to the pelvic floor muscle.

Yellow vessel loop indicated Hypogastric nerve from IHP

RECTOVAGINAL LIGAMENT DISSECTION, RIGHT
RIGHT EXTENDED PELVIC NODE DISSECTION

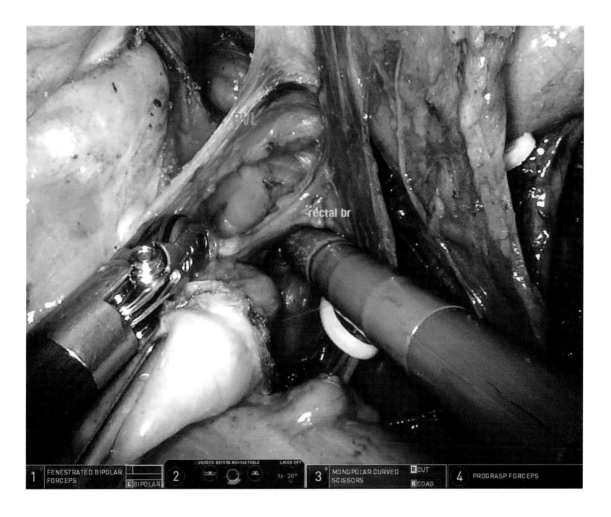

Fig. 42

The rectal branched of IHP was isolated from pelvic floor by the robotic Scissors

Rectal branches of IHP were communicated with Hypogastric nerve from IHP

Yellow vessel loop indicated Hypogastric nerve from IHP

Chapter 1

RECTOVAGINAL LIGAMENT DISSECTION, RIGHT
RIGHT EXTENDED PELVIC NODE DISSECTION

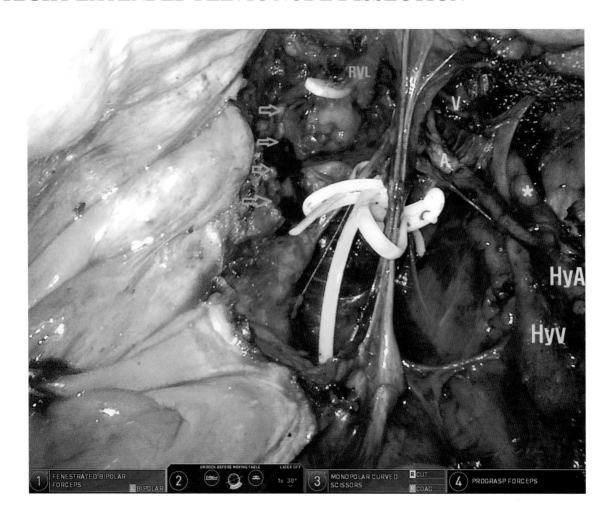

Fig. 43

After cutting the rectovaginal ligament, we can identify cut end of rectovaginal ligament, rectal part(green arrow) and vaginal part(RVL, hemo lok). rectal branches of inferior hypogastric plexus(blue vessel loop) and hypogastric nerve from inferior hypogastric plexus(yellow vessel loop), branches of pelvic splanchnic nerves which was not identified in this cases

• A(artery in the cardinal ligament)

• V(vein in the cardinal ligament)

* indicated anterior branches of hypogastric artery.

RECTOVAGINAL LIGAMENT DISSECTION, RIGHT
RIGHT EXTENDED PELVIC NODE DISSECTION

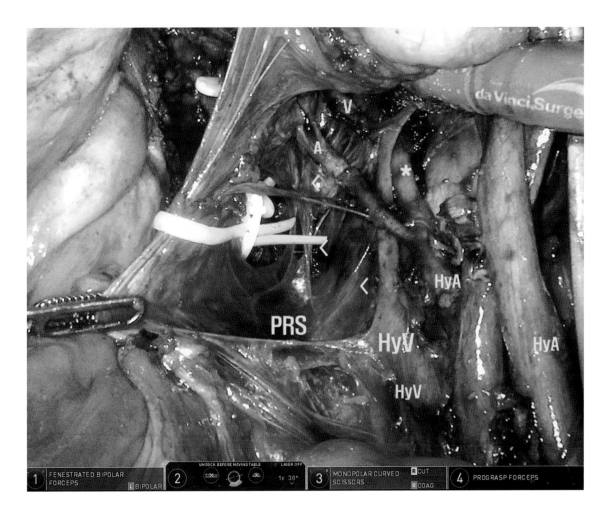

Fig. 44

Rectal branches of inferior hypogastric plexus(blue vessel loop) and hypogastric nerve from inferior hypogastric plexus (yellow vessel loop), branches of pelvic splanchnic nerves(PSN) which was identified after medial retraction of neural plane. PSN were located under the vessel.(<)

• PRS(pararectal space)

• A(artery in the cardinal ligament)

• V(vein in the cardinal ligament)

* indicated anterior branches of hypogastric artery.

Chapter 1

VESICOUTERINE LIGAMENT DISSECTION, RIGHT

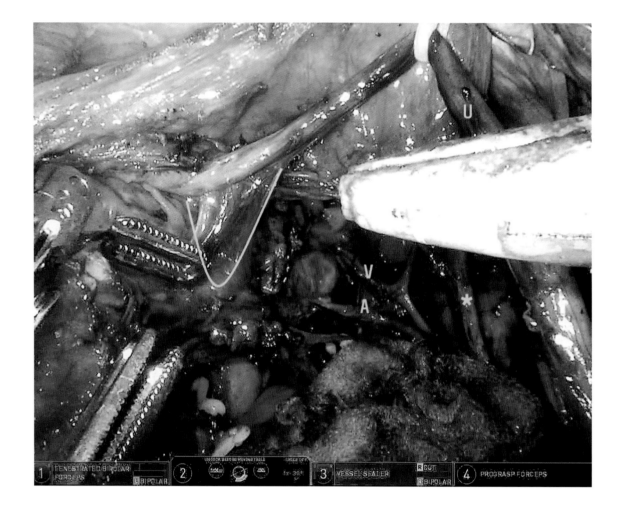

Fig. 45

After dissection of anterior vesicouterine ligament, we can identify the posterior vesicouterine ligament(v line). The tip of Bipolar grasp indicate the posterior vesicouterine ligament.

- A(artery in the cardinal ligament)
- V(vein in the cardinal ligament)
* indicated anterior branches of hypogastric artery.

VESICOUTERINE LIGAMENT DISSECTION, RIGHT

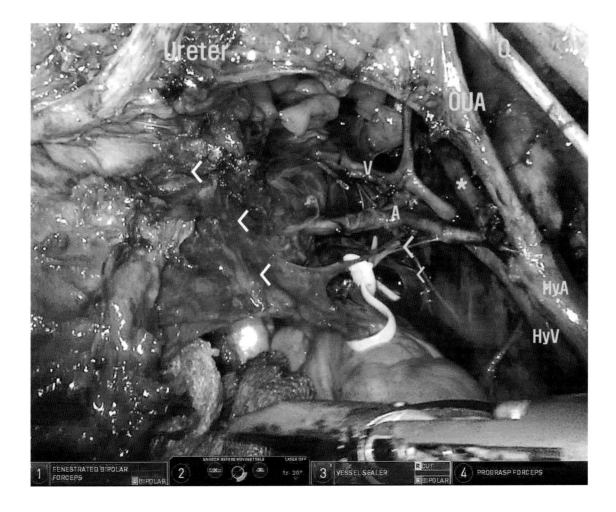

Fig. 46

This slide shows view of paravaginal tissue after complete cutting of post. Vesicouterine ligament, White < indicated vesical branches of IHP.
Yellow < indicated pelvic splanchnic nerves (PSN) which were located under the vessel

• A(artery in the cardinal ligament)

• V(vein in the cardinal ligament)

* indicated anterior branches of hypogastric artery.

Chapter 1

VESICOUTERINE LIGAMENT DISSECTION, RIGHT

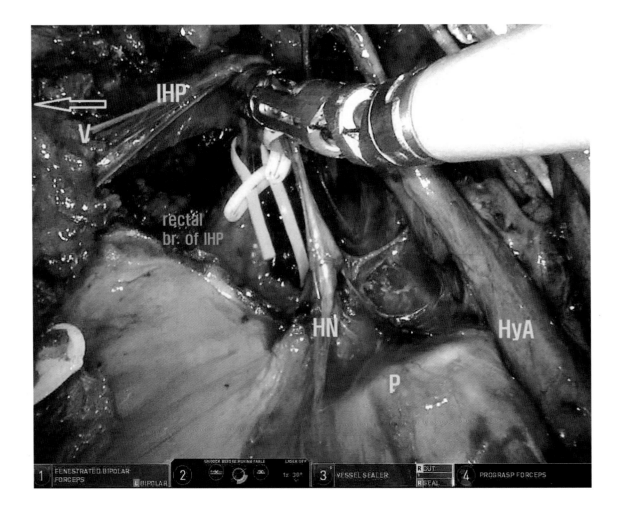

Fig. 47

This slide shows posterior of view of paravaginal tissue and neural tissues, rectal branches of inferior hypogastric plexus(blue vessel loop) and hypogastric nerve from inferior hypogastric plexus(yellow vessel loop).

- P(promontory)
- HyA(hypogastric artery)

Yellow arrow indicate the vesical branches of IHP.

PARAVAGINAL TISSUE DISSECTION, RIGHT

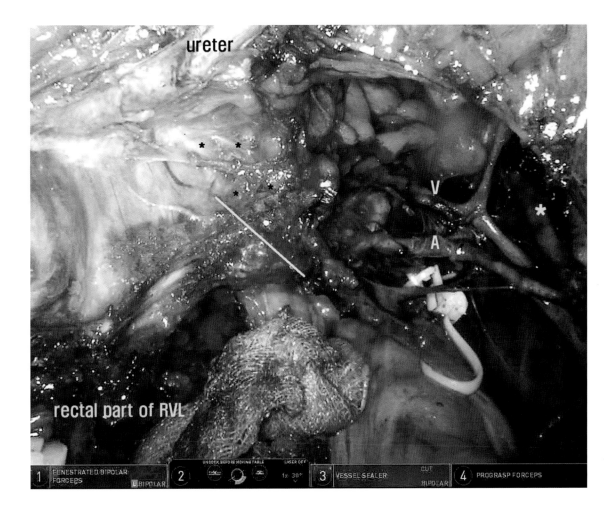

Fig. 48

This slide shows dissection line of paravaginal tissue(yellow line). And vesical branches of inferior hypogastric plexus(black*), rectal branches of inferior hypogastric plexus(blue vessel loop) and hypogastric nerve from inferior hypogastric plexus(yellow vessel loop).

• A(artery in the cardinal ligament)

• V(vein in the cardinal ligament)

• Yellow

* indicated anterior branches of hypogastric artery.

Chapter 1

PARAVAGINAL TISSUE DISSECTION, RIGHT

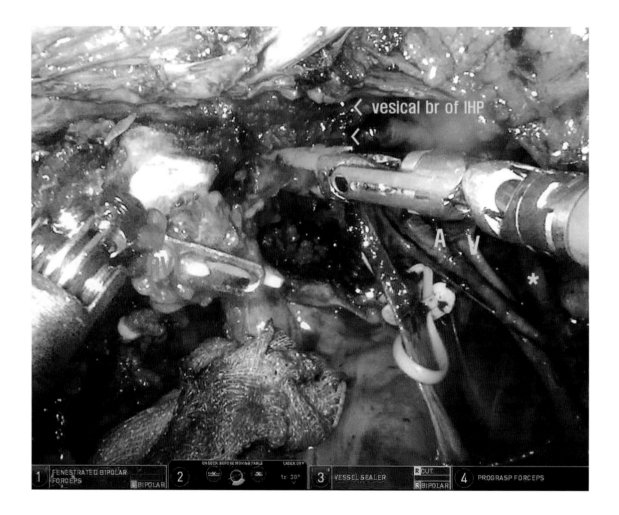

Fig. 49

This slide shows final dissection of paravaginal tissue by vessel sealer. In this point, it should not included the rectal branches of IHP or hypogastric nerve from IHP but should include vaginal part of rectovaginal ligament .

• A(artery in the cardinal ligament)

• V(vein in the cardinal ligament)

* indicated anterior branches of hypogastric artery.

EXTENDED PELVIC NODE DISSECTION, LEFT

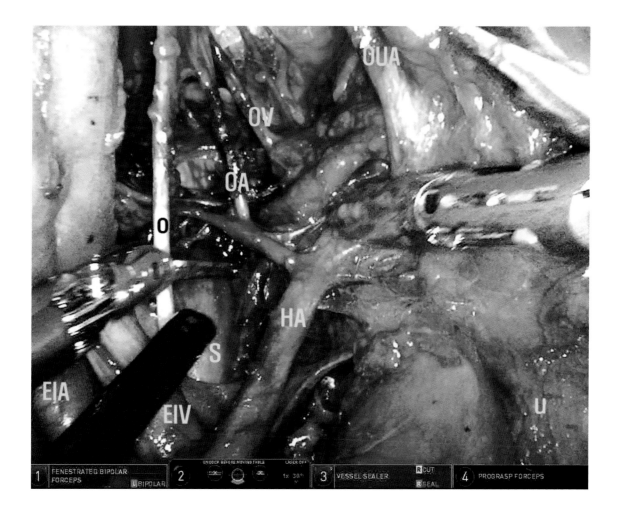

Fig. 50

This slide shows final dissection of left pelvic side.
The Superior and inferior gluteal artery were not seen in this slide.

- O(obturate nerve)
- S(sacral nerve)
- HA(hypogastric artery)
- OA(obturator artery)
- OV(obturator vein)

- EIA(external iliac artery)
- EIV(external iliac vein)
- U(ureter)
- OUA(obliterated umbilical artery)

Chapter 1

CARDINAL LIGAMENT DISSECTION, LEFT

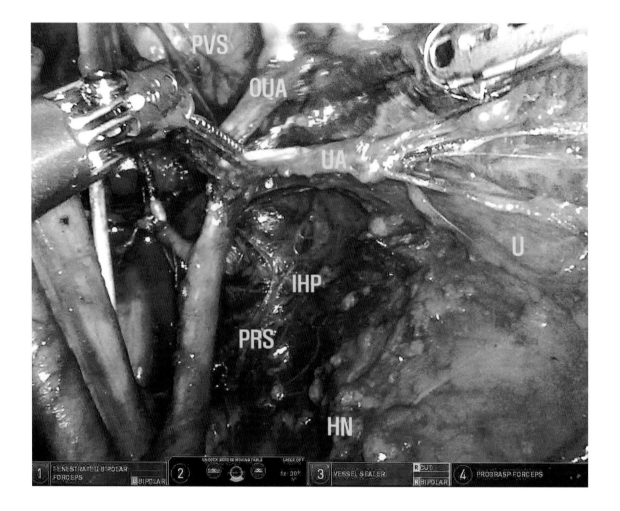

Fig. 51

Cardinal ligament which contained uterine artery (UA) and several branches of veins to the hypogastric vein was situated between the paravesical space (PVS) and pararectal space (PRS).

- OUA(obliterated umbilical artery)
- U(ureter)
- IHP(inferior hypogastric plexus)
- HN(hypogastric nerve)

CARDINAL LIGAMENT DISSECTION, LEFT

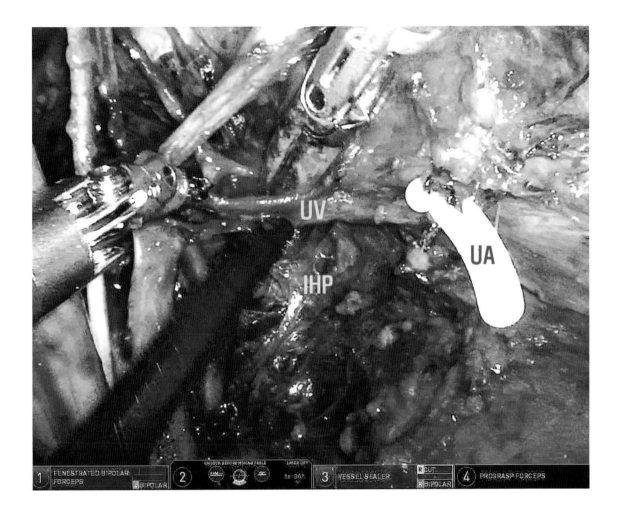

Fig. 52

After dividing uterine artery (UA), deep uterine vein(UV) were carefully isolated by vessel sealer and divided , at that time, be careful of Inferior hypogastric plexus(IHP) which was located under the vein, dorsomedial side.

Chapter 1

CARDINAL LIGAMENT DISSECTION, LEFT

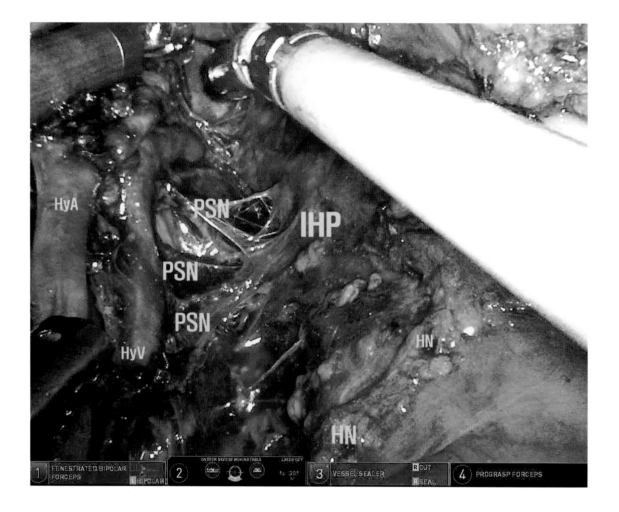

Fig. 53

After complete removal of uterine veins in cardinal ligament, we can identify anatomic communication of IHP with pelvic splanchnic nerves(PSN).
The tip of forceps were located at paravesical space.

• Hypogastric nerve(HN)
• HyA(hypogastric artery)
• HyV(hypogastric vein)

HN FROM IHP, LEFT

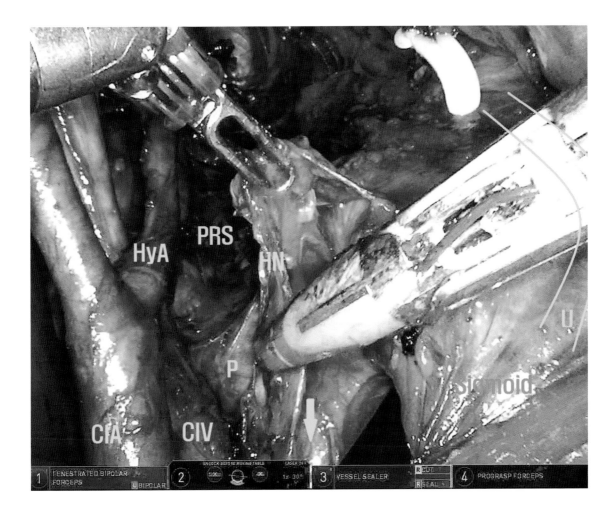

Fig. 54

After traction of hypogastric nerve by bipolar forceps, we identify the hypogastric nerve(HN) from superior hypogastric plexus(yellow arrow) At first we isolate left hypogastric nerve (HN) at level of left part of promontory (P), common iliac Vein(CIV) and common iliac artery(CIA). And we separate the hypogastric nerve from the IHP communicated with pelvic splanchnic nerves and separated from mesoureter plane to pelvic floor muscle completely.

- PRS(pararectal space)
- HyA(hypogastric artery)
- U(ureter)

Chapter 1

HN FROM IHP, LEFT

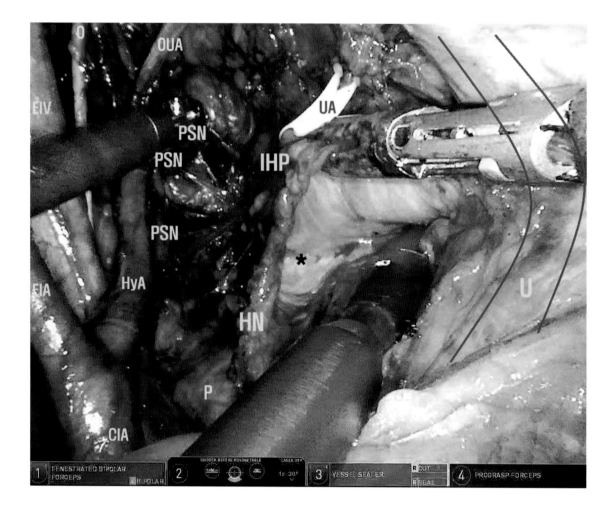

Fig. 55

After traction of hypogastric nerve by bipolar grasp, we identify the hypogastric nerve (HN) from superior hypogastric plexus (yellow arrow)

At first we isolate left hypogastric nerve (HN) at level of left part of promontory (P), common iliac Vein (CIV) and common iliac artery (CIA). And we separate the hypogastric nerve until the IHP communicated with pelvic splanchnic nerves and separated from mesoureter plane to pelvic floor completely.

* indicated pelvic floor muscle

- PRS(pararectal space)
- HyA(hypogastric artery)
- U(ureter)
- EIA(external iliac artery)

- OUA(obliterated umbilical artery)
- O(obturator nerve)
- UA(cut end of uterine artery),

HN FROM IHP, LEFT

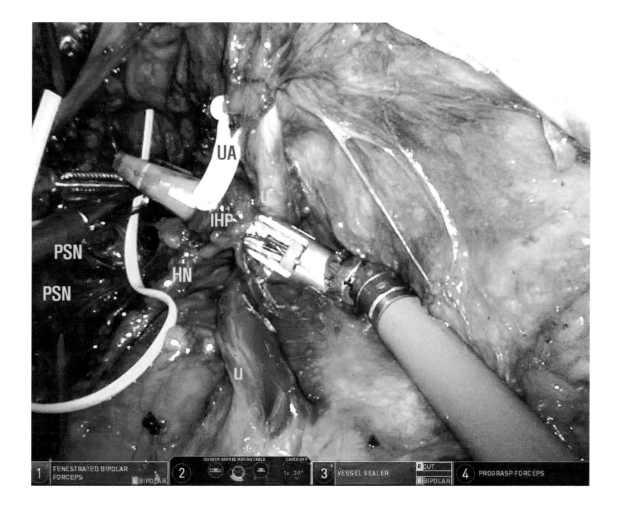

Fig. 56

We isolated IHP and hypogastric nerve by vessel sealer and marked with yellow vessel loop. This neural plane was rather firm and tense to perforate We can identify the level of anatomic plane from above were uterine artery, ureter, HN from IHP and PSN.

• PSN(pelvic splanchnic nerves)

• U(ureter)

Chapter 1

HN FROM IHP, LEFT

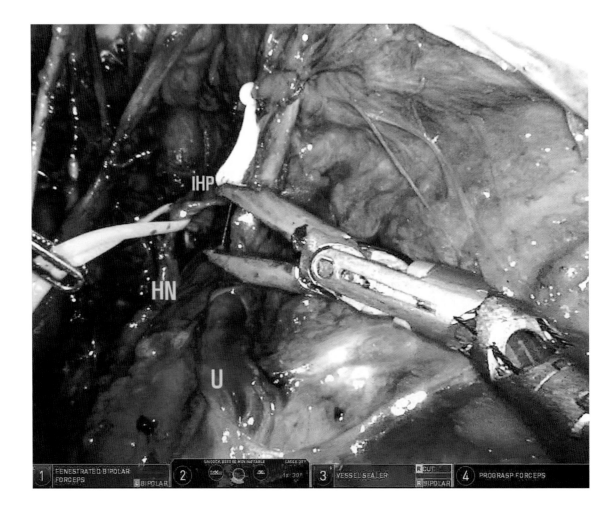

Fig. 57

We isolated hypogastric nerve from IHP with vessel sealer and marked with yellow vessel loop.

When we isolated and retracted hypogastric nerve from IHP by yellow vessel loop, we identified the anatomic relations in the pelvis

RESECTION OF RECTOVAGINAL LIGAMENT, LEFT

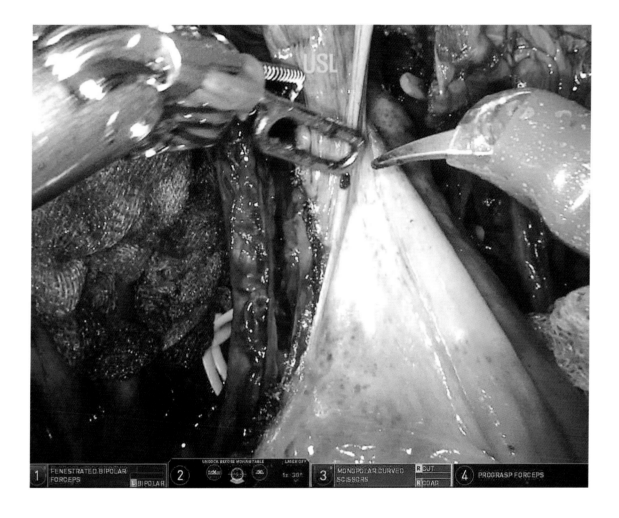

Fig. 58

After dissection of rectovaginal space, identify the rectum and pararectal space and medial border of rectovaginal ligament and uterosacral ligament. Yellow vessel loop indicated Hypogastric nerve from IHP.

Chapter 1

RESECTION OF RECTOVAGINAL LIGAMENT, LEFT

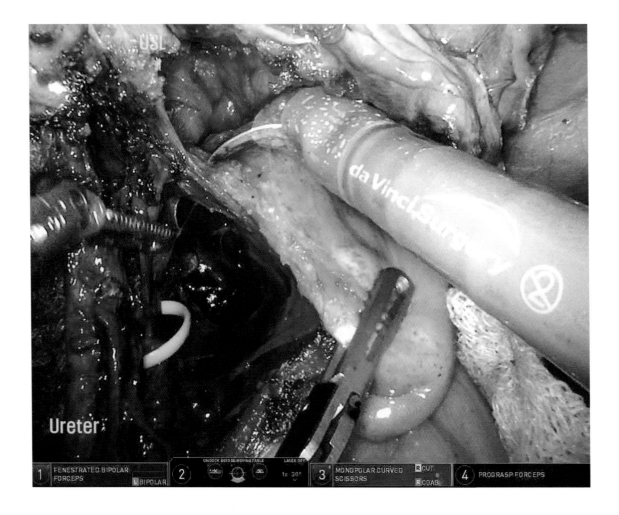

Fig. 59

After cutting the uterosacral ligament, we can identify medial and lateral margin of rectovaginal ligament, rectal branches of inferior hypogastric plexus(IHP) were located lateral border of rectovaginal ligament.

Tip of scissor indicated rectovaginal ligament which included rectal branches of IHP.

• USL(cut end of uterosacral ligament)

• HN from IHP(yellow vessel loop)

RESECTION OF RECTOVAGINAL LIGAMENT, LEFT

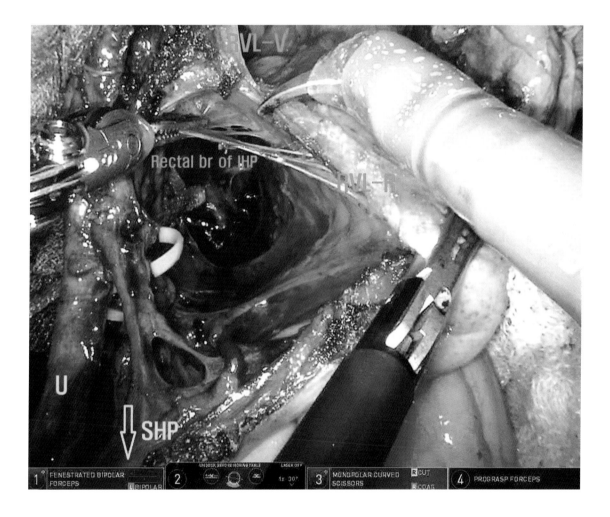

Fig. 60

We can separate the lateral situated rectal branches of IHP by sharp dissection.

Tip of scissor indicated rectal branches of IHP after superficial dissection of rectovaginal ligament.

- IHP and deep HN(yellow vessel loop)
- SHP(superficial hypogastric plexus)
- RVL-V(vaginal part of rectovaginal ligament)
- RVL-R(rectal part of rectovaginal ligament)

Chapter 1

RESECTION OF RECTOVAGINAL LIGAMENT, LEFT

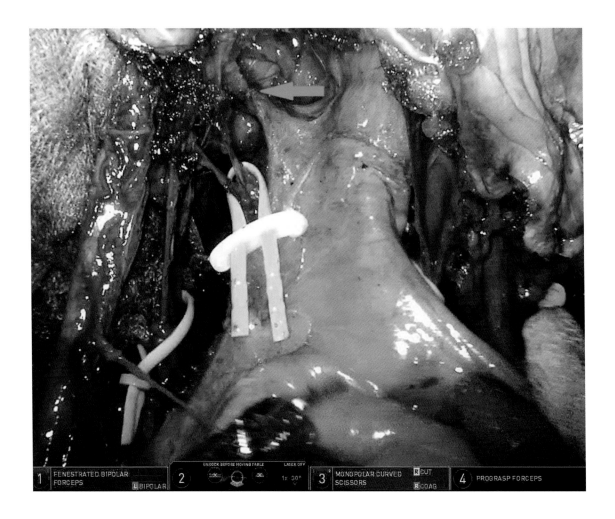

Fig. 61

We isolated the rectal branches of IHP by blue vessel loop.

Rectovaginal ligament(RVL) was not completely divided. (Green arrow)

• IHP and deep HN (yellow vessel loop)

RESECTION OF RECTOVAGINAL LIGAMENT, LEFT

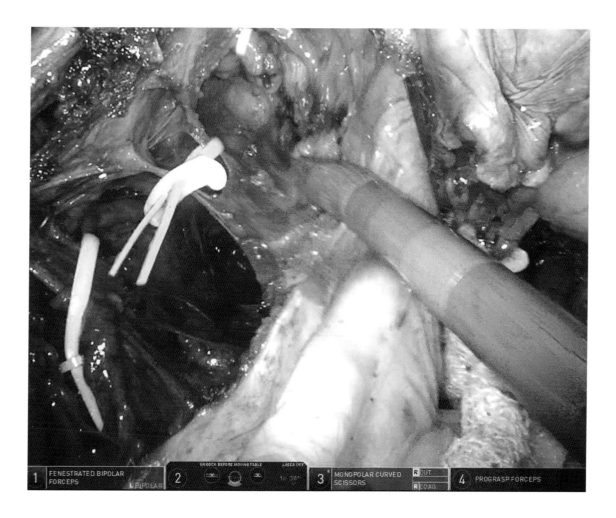

Fig. 62

We isolated the rectal branches of IHP by blue vessel loop.

Rectovaginal ligament was completely divided and vaginal end was marked with Hemo lok Inferior hypogastric plexus(IHP) and deep HN(yellow vessel loop), rectal branches of inferior hypogastric plexus (IHP) (blue vessel loop)

Chapter 1

RESECTION OF PARAVAGINAL TISSUE, LEFT

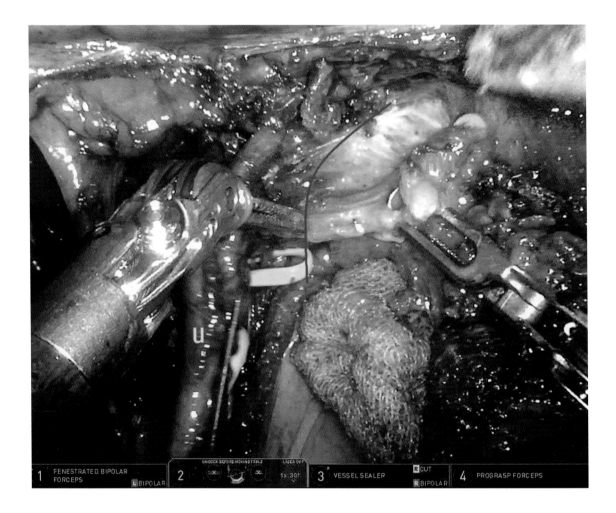

Fig. 63

Red line indicated resection line of paravaginal tissue under the cut end of rectovaginal ligament (RVL)
Inferior hypogastric plexus(IHP) and HN(yellow vessel loop), rectal branches of inferior hypogastric plexus (IHP) (blue vessel loop)

• U(ureter)

Case C (Fig. 64 – Fig. 98)

Conception of resection of rectovaginal ligament and preservation of rectal branches of inferior hypogastric plexus

Preservation of superior hypogastric plexus

Extended pelvic node dissection

Cardinal ligament dissection

Vesicouterine ligament dissection

Paravaginal dissection

For purpose of reducing local recurrence in the cervical cancer

Chapter 1

SUPERIOR HYPOGASTRIC PLEXUS

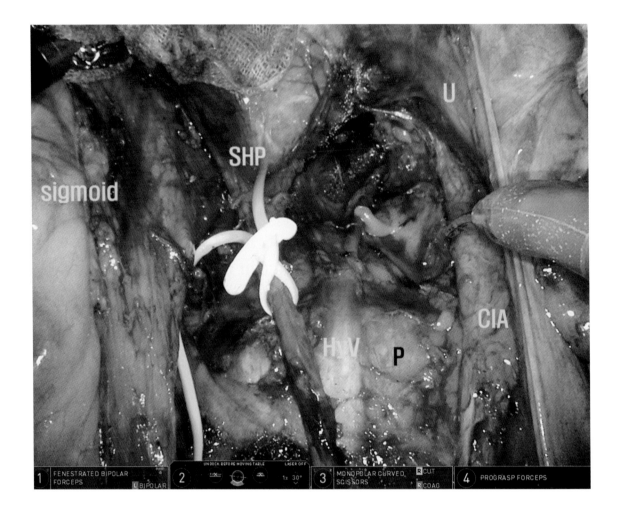

Fig. 64

Superior hypogastric plexus(SHP)was isolated by long yellow vessel loop

- U(ureter)
- P(promontory)
- HyV(hypogastric vein anomaly)
- CIA(common iliac artery)

RIGHT EXTENDED PELVIC NODE DISSECTION

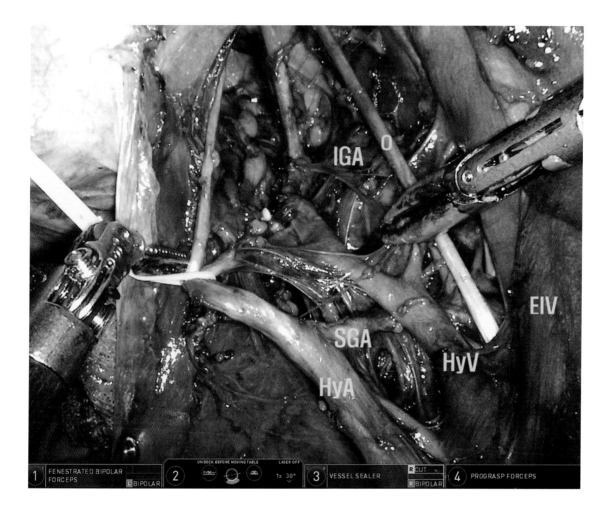

Fig. 65

In this case, the vessel pattern were more complicated.
To dissect more extensively, we used vessel sealer instrument and divided the vessel without excessive bleeding .

Nodes were removed by pulling the tissue by tip of bipolar or vessel sealer

- IGA(inferior gluteal artery)
- SGA(superior gluteal artery)
- SGV(superior gluteal vein)
- OUA(obliterated umbilical artery)
- O(obtrurator nerve)

- EIA(external iliac artery)
- EIV(external iliac vein)
- HyA(hypogastric artery)
- HyV(hypogastric vein)

Chapter 1

RIGHT EXTENDED PELVIC NODE DISSECTION

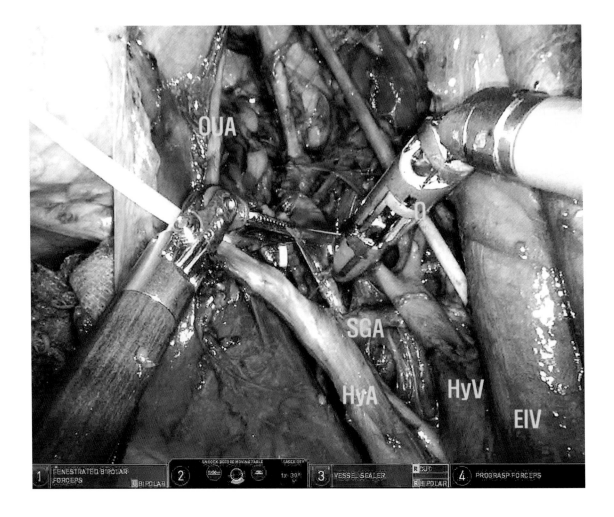

Fig. 66

In this case, there was more complicated vessel To dissect more extensively or to identify the deep structures, we used vessel sealer instrument and sealed and cut the veins without excessive bleeding .

- IGA (inferior gluteal artery)
- SGA (superior gluteal artery)
- SGV (superior gluteal vein)
- OUA (obliterated umbilical artery)
- O (obtrurator nerve)
- EIA (external iliac artery)
- EIV (external iliac vein)

- HyA (hypogastric artery)
- HyV (hypogastric vein)
- EIA(external iliac artery)
- EIV(external iliac vein)
- HyA(hypogastric artery)
- HyV(hypogastric vein)

RIGHT EXTENDED PELVIC NODE DISSECTION

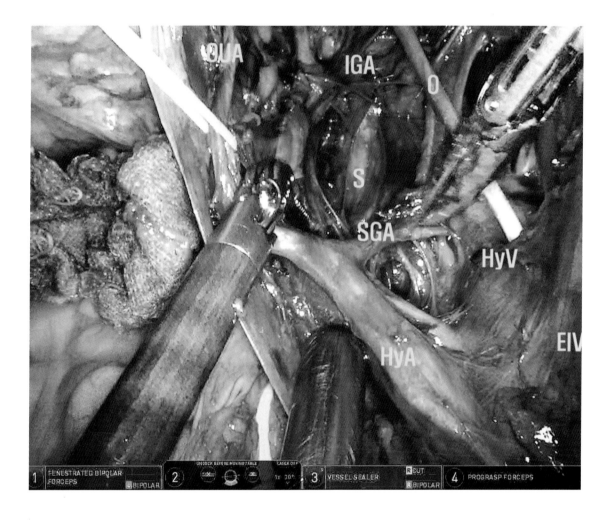

Fig. 67

After removal of branches of veins, we identify the sacral nerves, IGA and SGA.

- IGA (inferior gluteal artery)
- SGA(superior gluteal artery)
- SGV (superior gluteal vein)
- OUA (obliterated umbilical artery)
- O (obtrurator nerve)

- EIA(external iliac artery)
- EIV(external iliac vein)
- HyA(hypogastric artery)
- HyV(hypogastric vein)
- S(sacral nerve)

Chapter 1

CARDINAL LIGAMENT DISSECTION, RIGHT

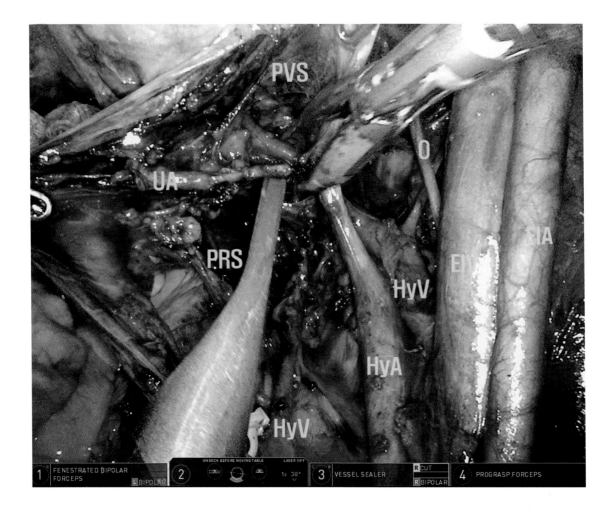

Fig. 68

Cardinal ligament which contained uterine artery (UA) and several branches of veins to the hypogastric vein was situated between the paravesical space (PVS) and pararectal space (PRS). Uterine artery was divided by vessel sealer ad distal part was marked by hemo lok

- IGA(inferior gluteal artery)
- SGA(superior gluteal artery)
- SGV(superior gluteal vein)
- OUA(obliterated umbilical artery)
- O(obtrurator nerve)
- EIA(external iliac artery)
- EIV(external iliac vein)
- HyA(hypogastric artery)
- HyV(hypogastric vein)
- EIA(external iliac artery)
- EIV(external iliac vein)
- HyA(hypogastric artery)
- HyV(hypogastric vein)
- S(sacral nerve)

CARDINAL LIGAMENT DISSECTION, RIGHT

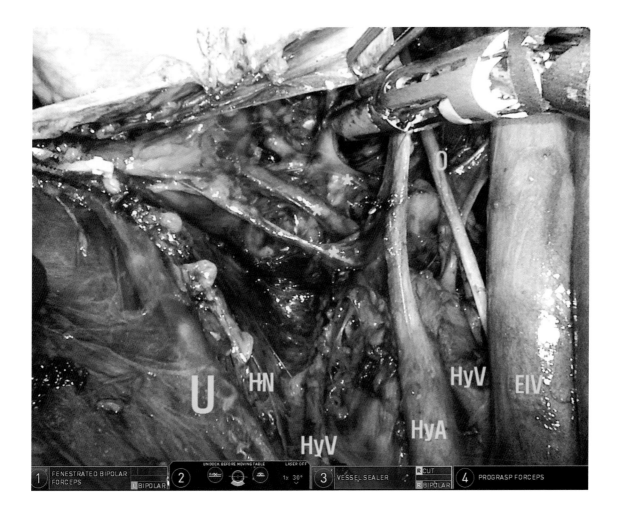

Fig. 69

In this case, there were several veins(*) in the cardinal ligament which were Sealed and divided by vessel sealer instrument.

- IGA(inferior gluteal artery)
- SGA(superior gluteal artery)
- SGV(superior gluteal vein)
- OUA(obliterated umbilical artery)
- O(obtrurator nerve)

- EIA(external iliac artery)
- EIV(external iliac vein)
- HyA(hypogastric artery)
- HyV(hypogastric vein)

Chapter 1

CARDINAL LIGAMENT DISSECTION, RIGHT

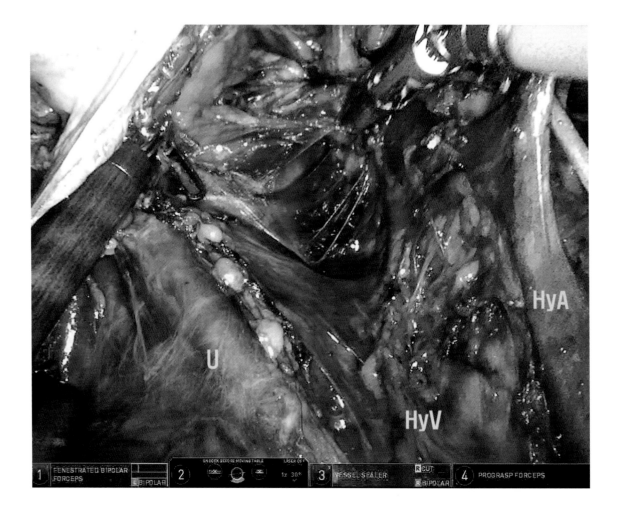

Fig. 70

This slide showed post operative complete dissection of cardinal ligament .

- IGA(inferior gluteal artery)
- SGA(superior gluteal artery)
- SGV(superior gluteal vein)
- OUA(obliterated umbilical artery)
- O(obtrurator nerve)

- EIA(external iliac artery)
- EIV(external iliac vein)
- HyA(hypogastric artery)
- HyV(hypogastric vein)
- U(ureter)

CARDINAL LIGAMENT DISSECTION, RIGHT

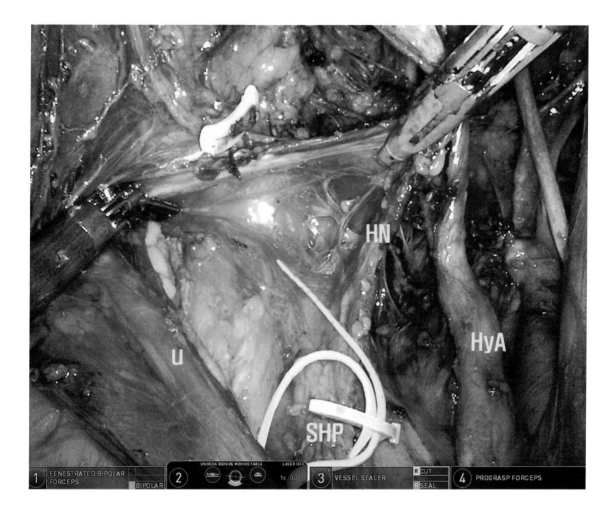

Fig. 71

Hypogastric nerve from IHP(Neural plane) were separated from mesoureter plane to the pelvic floor.

Hypogastric nerve was communicated with SHP (long yellow vessel loop) from above.

- IGA (inferior gluteal artery)
- SGA (superior gluteal artery)
- SGV (superior gluteal vein)
- OUA (obliterated umbilical artery)
- O(obtrurator nerve)
- EIA (external iliac artery)

- EIV (external iliac vein)
- HyA (hypogastric artery)
- HyV(hypogastric vein)
- U (ureter)
- SHP (superior hypogastric plexus)

Chapter 1

CARDINAL LIGAMENT DISSECTION, RIGHT

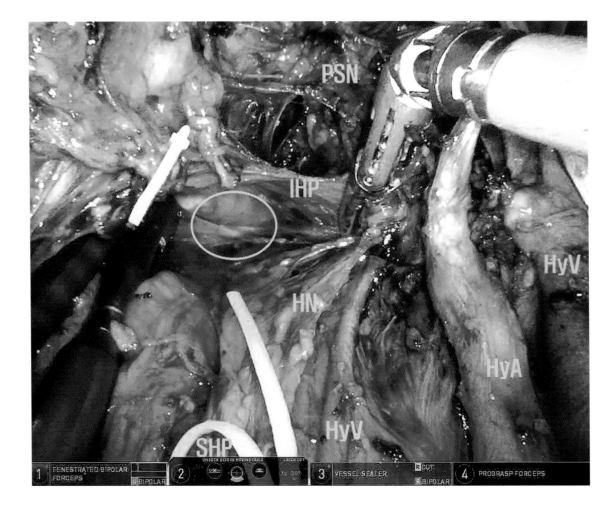

Fig. 72

Hypogastric nerve from IHP(Neural plane) were separated from mesoureter plane to the pelvic floor muscle. Round circle area was Okabayashi space.

- IGA(inferior gluteal artery)
- SGA(superior gluteal artery)
- SGV(superior gluteal vein)
- OUA(obliterated umbilical artery)
- O(obtrurator nerve)
- EIA(external iliac artery)

- EIV(external iliac vein)
- HyA(hypogastric artery)
- PSN(pelvic splanchnic nerves)
- HyV(hypogastric vein)
- U(ureter)

CARDINAL LIGAMENT DISSECTION, RIGHT

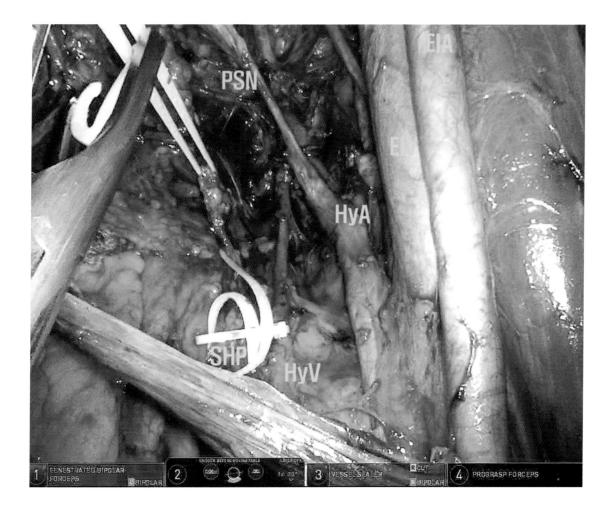

Fig. 73

Hypogastric nerve from IHP (Neural plane) were isolated from mesoureter plane down to the pelvic floor (yellow vessel loop). These nerves were isolated from pelvic floor. This neural plane was rather thick and firm to perforate. In these thick, firm neural plane can protect the local lateral spread of cancer.

- IGA(inferior gluteal artery)
- SGA(superior gluteal artery)
- SGV(superior gluteal vein)
- OUA(obliterated umbilical artery)
- O(obtrurator nerve)
- EIA(external iliac artery)

- EIV(external iliac vein)
- HyA(hypogastric artery)
- PSN(pelvic splanchnic nerves)
- HyV(hypogastric vein)
- U (ureter)

Chapter 1

LEFT EXTENDED PELVIC NODE DISSECTION

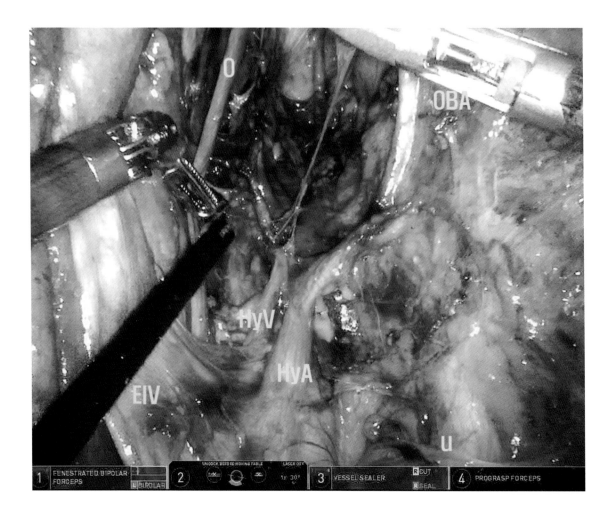

Fig. 74

In this case, there was rather simple vascular structure.

To dissect more extensively, we used vessel sealer instrument and divided the vein without excessive bleeding .

- IGA(inferior gluteal artery)
- SGA(superior gluteal artery)
- SGV(superior gluteal vein)
- OUA(obliterated umbilical artery)
- O(obtrurator nerve)

- EIA(external iliac artery)
- EIV(external iliac vein)
- HyA(hypogastric artery)
- HyV(hypogastric vein)

LEFT EXTENDED PELVIC NODE DISSECTION

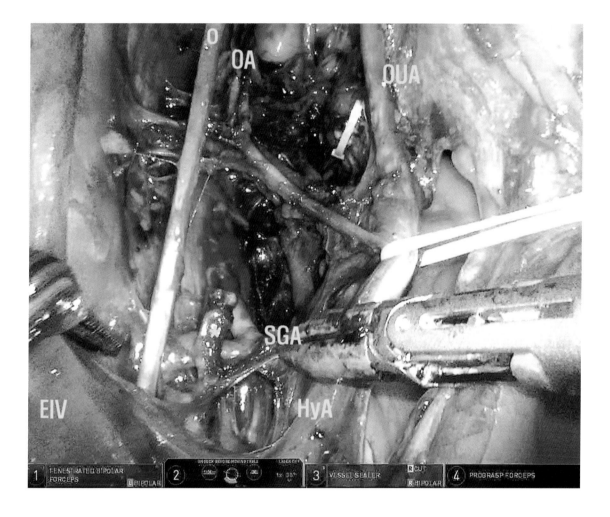

Fig. 75

After dividing the hypogastric vein(*). we can identify the deep structures, such as SGA, S1(sacral nerve 1st), LST (lumbosacral trunk)

- IGA(inferior gluteal artery)
- SGA(superior gluteal artery)
- SGV(superior gluteal vein)
- OUA(obliterated umbilical artery)
- O(obtrurator nerve)

- OA(obturator artery)
- EIA(external iliac artery)
- EIV(external iliac vein)
- HyA(hypogastric artery)
- HyV(hypogastric vein)

Chapter 1

CARDINAL LIGAMENT DISSECTION, LEFT

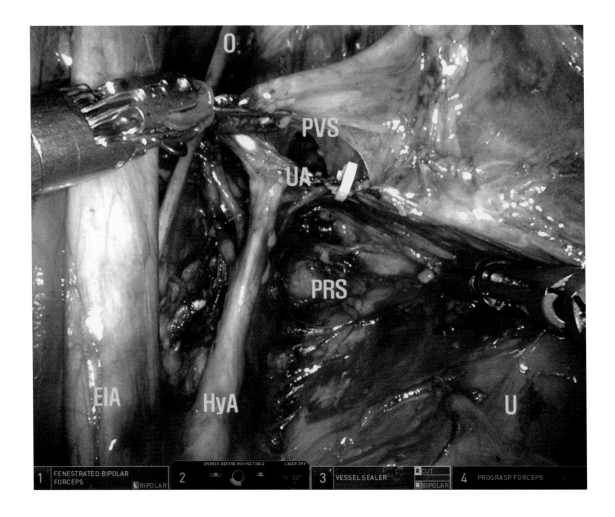

Fig. 76

Cardinal ligament which contained uterine artery (UA) and several branches of veins to hypogastric vein was situated between the paravesical space (PVS) and pararectal space (PRS).

- OUA(obliterated umbilical artery)
- U(ureter)
- IHP(inferior hypogastric plexus)
- HN(hypogastric nerve)

CARDINAL LIGAMENT DISSECTION, LEFT

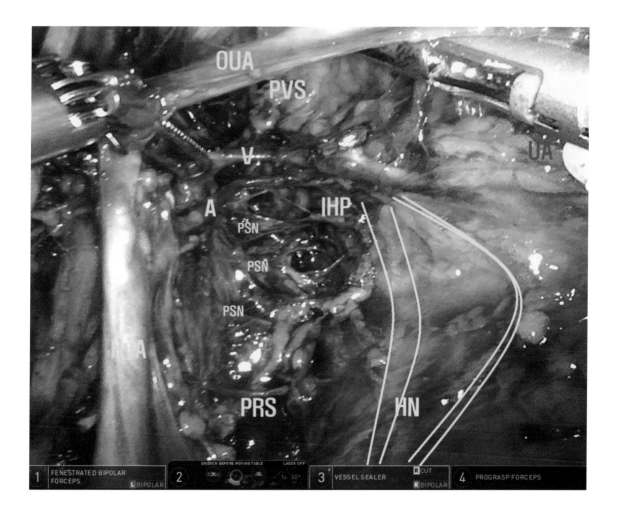

Fig. 77

There were anatomic relationship with PSN , IHP, HN and vessel in cardinal ligament.

- OUA(obliterated umbilical artery)
- U(ureter)
- IHP(inferior hypogastric plexus)
- HN(hypogastric nerve)

- V(deep uterine vein)
- PSN(pelvic splanchnic nerves)
- A(anomaly artery)

Chapter 1

CARDINAL LIGAMENT DISSECTION, LEFT

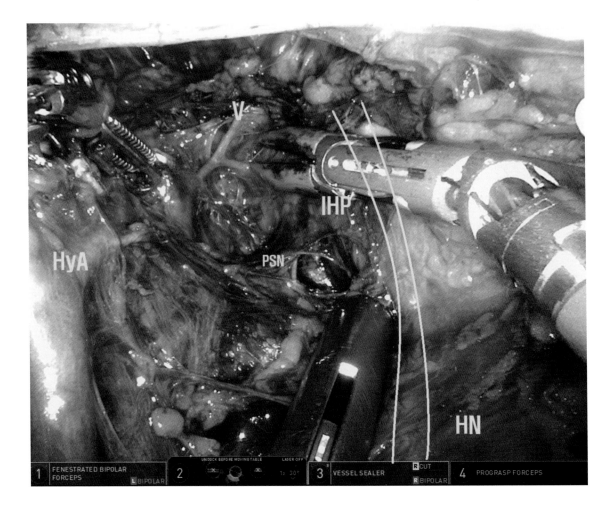

Fig. 78

Paravesical space and pararectal space was communicated after dividing the vessel of cardinal ligament.

Cardinal ligament which contained uterine artery (UA) and several branches of veins to hypogastric vein was situated between the paravesical space (PVS) and pararectal space (PRS)

- OUA(obliterated umbilical artery)
- U (ureter)
- IHP(inferior hypogastric plexus)

- HN (hypogastric nerve)
- V(deep uterine vein)

CARDINAL LIGAMENT DISSECTION, LEFT

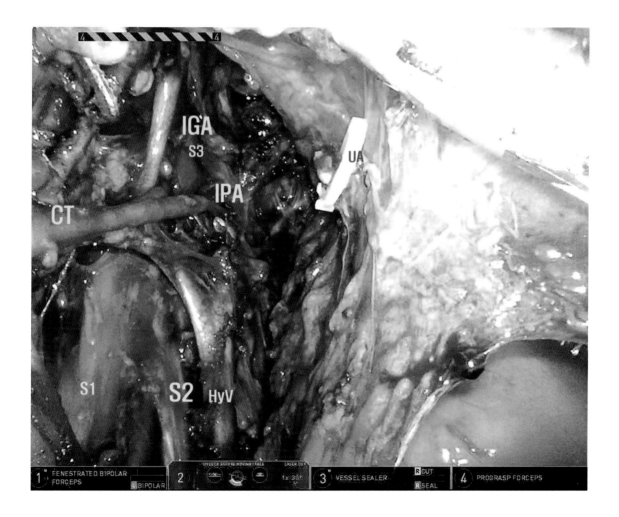

Fig. 79

CT(common trunk) of IGA(inferior gluteal artery) and IPA(internal pudendal artery) S1(sacral nerve 1st), S2(sacral nerve 2nd), S3(sacral nerve 3rd).

• HyV(hypogastric vein)

Chapter 1

CARDINAL LIGAMENT DISSECTION, LEFT

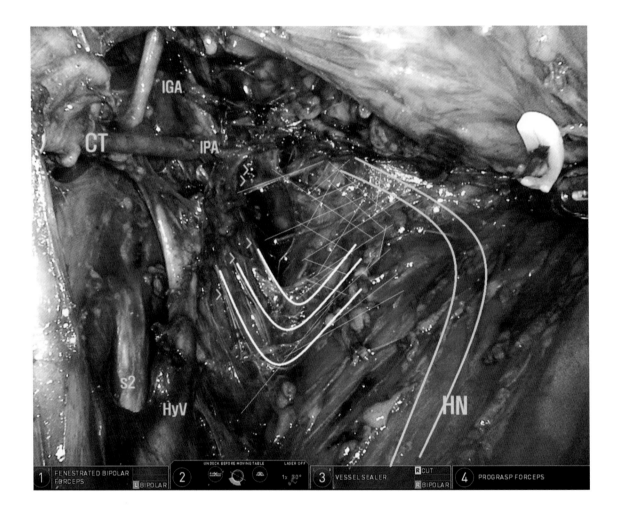

Fig. 80

Paravesical space and pararectal space was communicated after dividing the vessel of cardinal ligament.

PSN (pelvic splanchnic nerve) were identified as thin multiple web like structures in the pararectal space (white lines) Hypogastric nerves were indicated as double yellow lines.

CT(common trunk) of IGA(inferior gluteal artery) and IPA(internal pudendal artery)

S2(sacral nerve 2nd)

S3(sacral nerve 3rd)

HN FROM IHP, LEFT

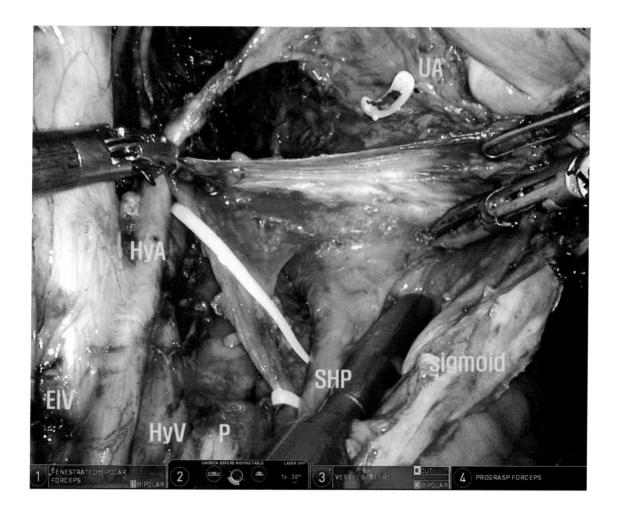

Fig. 81

Hypogastric nerve(HN) was communicated with SHP from above. We can identify the HN more easily because of HN was downward branches of SHP
Neural plane(hypogastric nerve from IHP) were separated from mesoureter plane to the pelvic floor muscle.

- IGA(inferior gluteal artery)
- SGA(superior gluteal artery)
- SGV(superior gluteal vein)
- OUA(obliterated umbilical artery)
- O(obturator nerve)
- EIA(external iliac artery)

- EIV(external iliac vein)
- HyA(hypogastric artery)
- HyV(hypogastric vein)
- U(ureter)
- SHP(superior hypogastric plexus)

Chapter 1

HN FROM IHP, LEFT

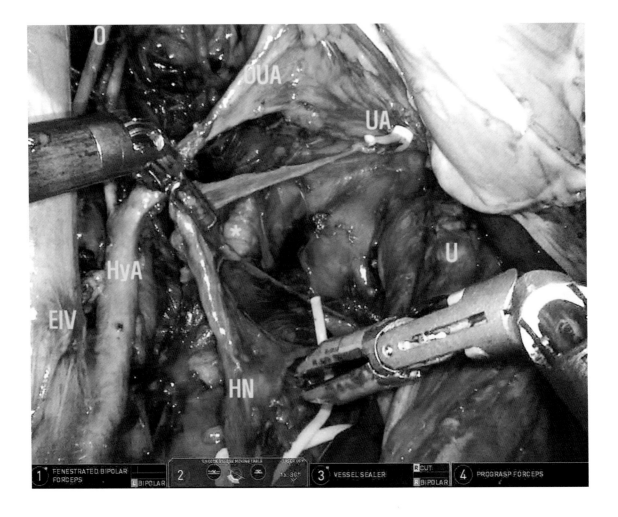

Fig. 82

Hypogastric nerve(HN) was communicated with SHP(long yellow vessel loop) from above. We can identify the HN more easily because of HN was downward branches of SHP Neural plane(hypogastric nerve from IHP) were separated from mesoureter plane to the pelvic floor muscle.(*)

- IGA(inferior gluteal artery)
- SGA(superior gluteal artery)
- SGV(superior gluteal vein)
- OUA(obliterated umbilical artery)
- O(obrrurator nerve)
- EIA(external iliac artery)
- EIV(external iliac vein)
- HyA(hypogastric artery)
- HyV(hypogastric vein)
- U(ureter)
- SHP(superior hypogastric plexus)

HN FROM IHP, LEFT

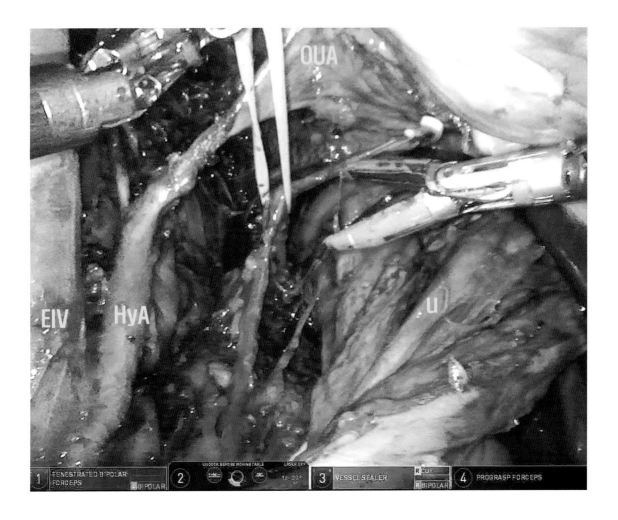

Fig. 83

HN from IHP were isolated with yellow vessel loop.

- IGA(inferior gluteal artery)
- SGA(superior gluteal artery)
- SGV(superior gluteal vein)
- OUA(obliterated umbilical artery)
- O(obtrurator nerve)
- EIA(external iliac artery)

- EIV(external iliac vein)
- HyA(hypogastric artery)
- HyV(hypogastric vein)
- U(ureter)
- SHP(superior hypogastric plexus)

Chapter 1

RECTOVAGINAL LIGAMENT DISSECTION, RIGHT
RIGHT EXTENDED PELVIC NODE DISSECTION

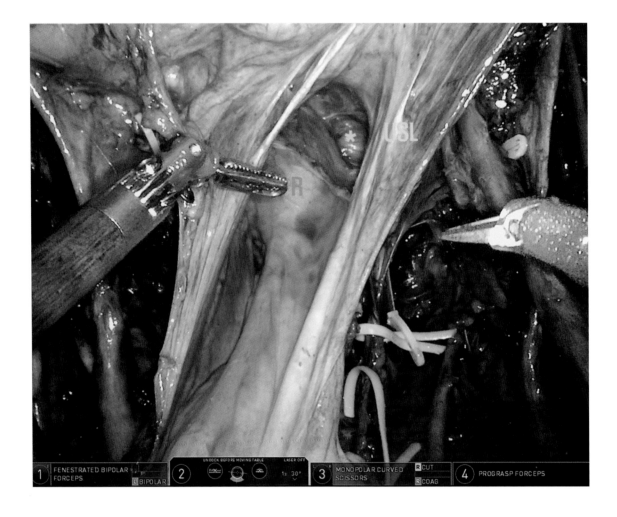

Fig. 84

After dissection of rectovaginal space, identify the rectum and pararectal space and medial border of rectovaginal ligament and uterosacral ligament. then cut uterosacral ligament and identify the rectovaginal ligament .

RECTOVAGINAL LIGAMENT DISSECTION, RIGHT
RIGHT EXTENDED PELVIC NODE DISSECTION

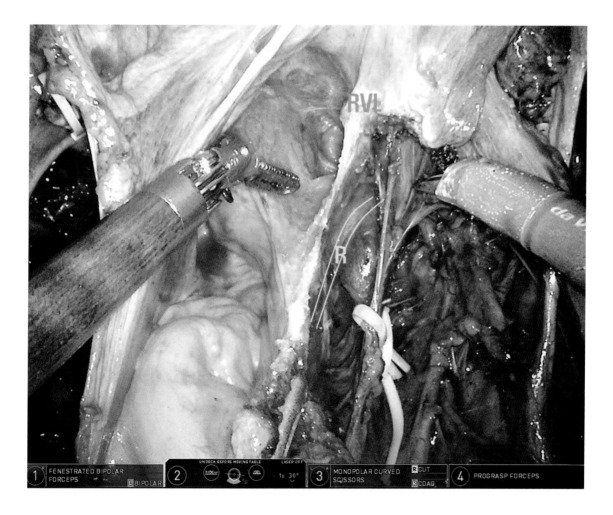

Fig. 85

After dissection of rectovaginal space, identify the rectum and pararectal space and medial border of rectovaginal ligament and uterosacral ligament. hen cut uterosacral ligament and identify the rectovaginal ligament (RVL) which located deeper than the IHP and HN (yellow vessel loop)

R– rectal branches of IHP which located lateral border of RVL

Yellow vessel loop indicated Hypogastric nerve and IHP

Chapter 1

RECTOVAGINAL LIGAMENT DISSECTION, RIGHT RIGHT EXTENDED PELVIC NODE DISSECTION

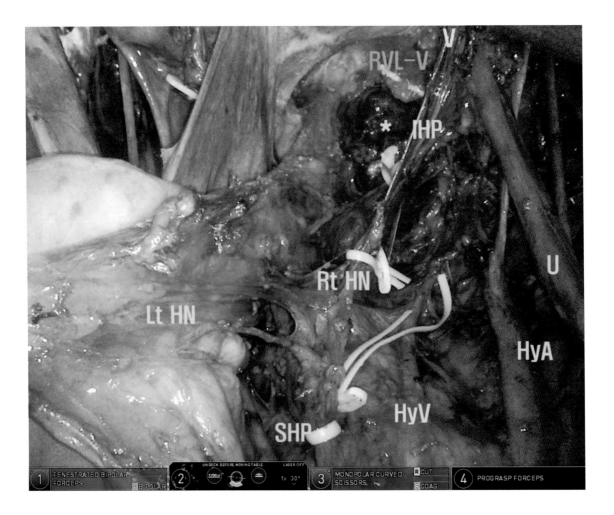

Fig. 86

Schematic Fig.ure of SHP to left and right HN and rectal branches of IHP(inferior hypogastric plexus) an pelvic splanchnic nerves (PSN) and vesical branches of IHP (V)

* indicate pelvic floor

• RVL-V(cur end of vaginal part of rectovaginal ligament)

• HyA(hypogastric artery)

• U(ureter)

RECTOVAGINAL LIGAMENT DISSECTION, LEFT RIGHT EXTENDED PELVIC NODE DISSECTION

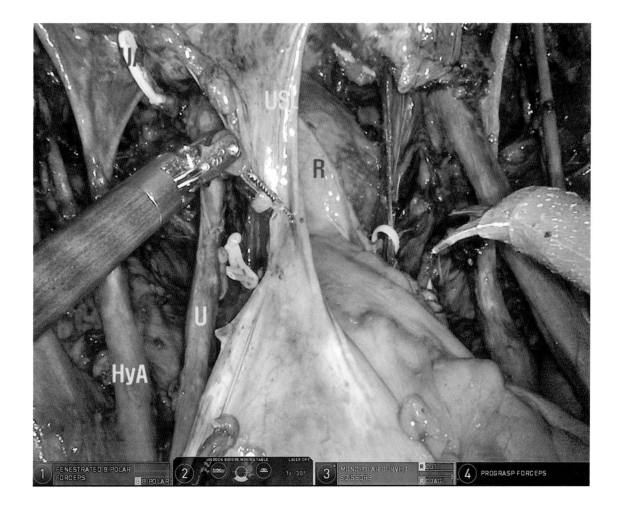

Fig. 87

After dissection of rectovaginal space, identify the rectum and pararectal space and medial border of rectovaginal ligament and uterosacral ligament. Yellow vessel loop indicated Hypogastric nerve and IHP.

• HyA (hypogastric artery)

Chapter 1

RECTOVAGINAL LIGAMENT DISSECTION, LEFT RIGHT EXTENDED PELVIC NODE DISSECTION

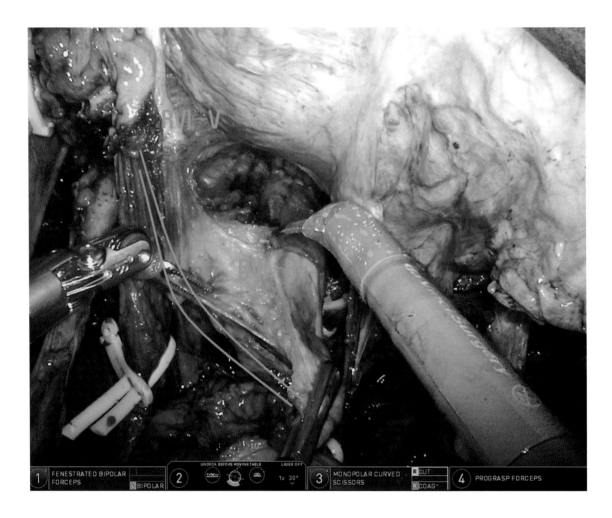

Fig. 88

After cutting the uterosacral ligament, we can identify medial and lateral margin of rectovaginal ligament, rectal branches of inferior hypogastric plexus(IHP) were located lateral border of rectovaginal ligament.(double green lines)

Next procedures were to separate the rectal branches of IHP from RVL by robotic scissors.

- RVL-R(rectal part of rectovaginal ligament)
- RVL-V(vaginal part of rectovaginal ligament)
- HN from IHP(yellow vessel loop)

RECTOVAGINAL LIGAMENT DISSECTION, LEFT RIGHT EXTENDED PELVIC NODE DISSECTION

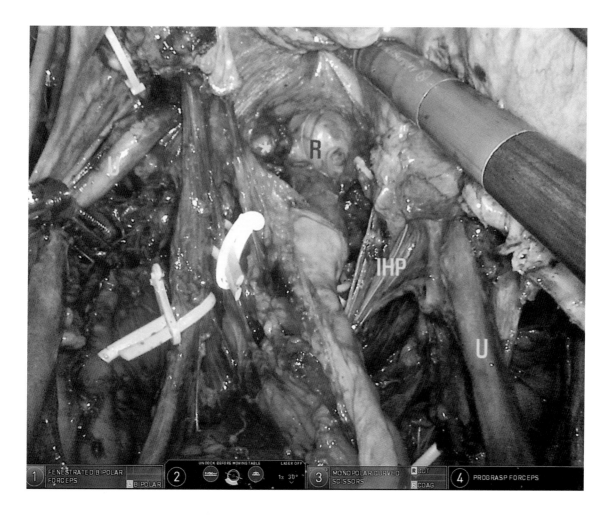

Fig. 89

We isolated the rectal branches of IHP by blue vessel loop.

Rectovaginal ligament was not completely divided Inferior hypogastric plexus(IHP) and deep HN(yellow vessel loop), rectal branches of inferior hypogastric plexus(IHP) (blue vessel loop)

* indicated pelvic floor muscle

Chapter 1

RECTOVAGINAL LIGAMENT DISSECTION, LEFT RIGHT EXTENDED PELVIC NODE DISSECTION

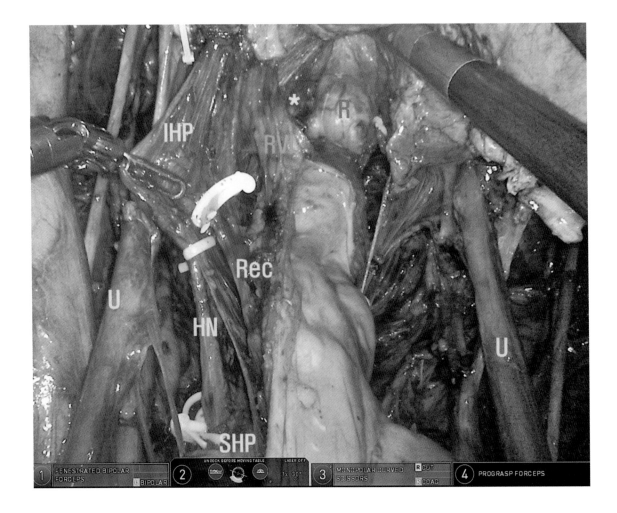

Fig. 90

This slide showed communication of SHP and HN, HP rand rectal braches of IHP (Rec).
We isolated the rectal branches of IHP by blue vessel loop.

Rectovaginal ligament was not completely divided Inferior hypogastric plexus(IHP) and deep HN(yellow vessel loop), Rec-(rectal branches of inferior hypogastric plexus (IHP) (blue vessel loop)

* indicated pelvic floor muscle

VESICOUTERINE LIGAMENT, RIGHT

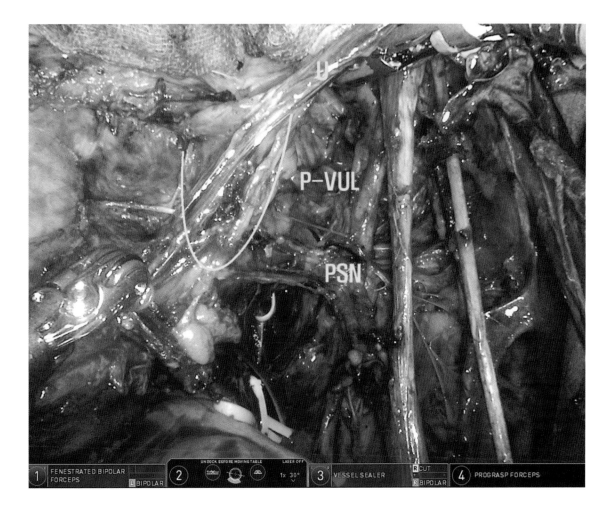

Fig. 91

This slide showed posterior vesicouterine ligament We can identify the anatomic relation with PSN and Rectal branches od IHP, HN from IHP. PSN(pelvic splanchnic nerves)

Inferior hypogastric plexus(IHP) and deep HN (yellow vessel loop), REC-rectal branches of inferior hypogastric plexus (IHP) (blue vessel loop)

Chapter 1

VESICOUTERINE LIGAMENT, RIGHT

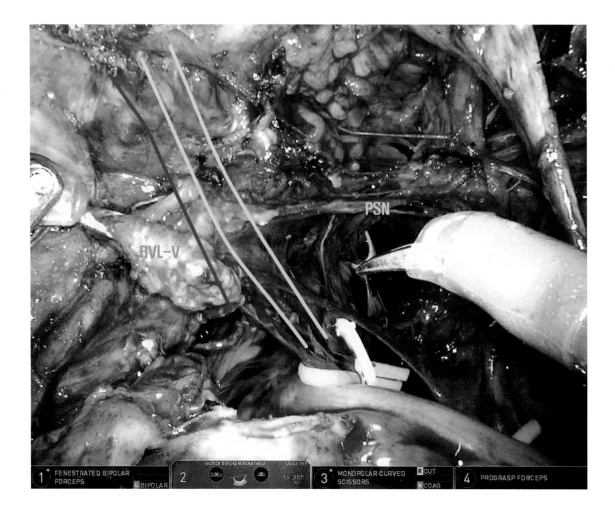

Fig. 92

Red line indicated the resection line of paravaginal tissue. Yellow line indicated the vesical branches of IHP

We could find the anatomic neural structures more exatly. PSN(pelvic splanchnic nerves)
Inferior hypogastric plexus(IHP) and deep HN(yellow vessel loop), RVL-V(cut end of vaginal part of rectovaginal ligament) REC-rectal branches of inferior hypogastric plexus(IHP) (blue vessel loop)

VESICOUTERINE LIGAMENT, RIGHT

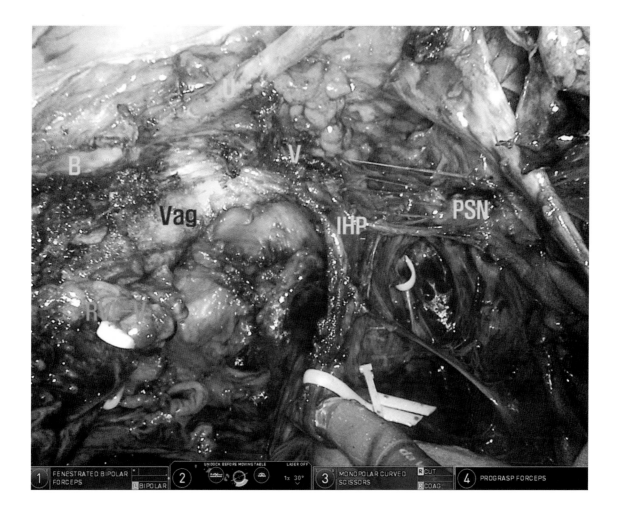

Fig. 93

This slide showed complete resection of posterior vesicouterine ligament. and resection of paravaginal tissue .

We can identify the anatomic relation with PSN and Rectal branches od IHP, HN from IHP. And vagina and vaginal part of Rectovaginal ligament.(RVL-V)

• PSN(pelvic splanchnic nerves)

• V(vesical branches of IHP)

Inferior hypogastric plexus(IHP) and deep HN(yellow vessel loop), rectal branches of inferior hypogastric plexus (IHP) (blue vessel loop)

Chapter 1

VESICOUTERINE LIGAMENT, LEFT

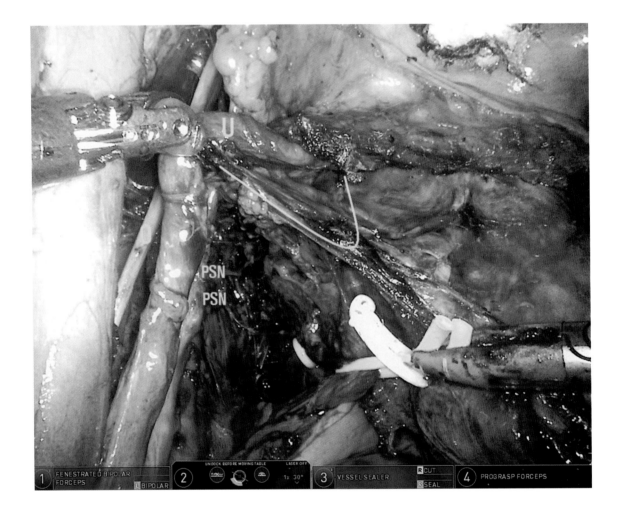

Fig. 94

This slide showed posterior vesicouterine ligament. (yellow line) We can identify the anatomic relation with PSN, Rectal branches od IHP and HN from IHP.

• PSN(pelvic splanchnic nerves)

• V(vesical branches of IHP)

Inferior hypogastric plexus(IHP) and deep HN(yellow vessel loop), REC-rectal branches of inferior hypogastric plexus (IHP) (blue vessel loop)

VESICOUTERINE LIGAMENT, LEFT

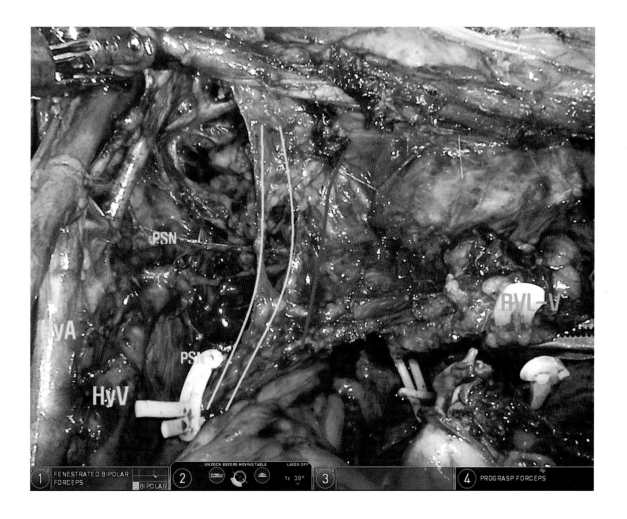

Fig. 95

This slide showed resection line of paravaginal tissue (red line) Yellow line indicated vesical branches of IHP

We can identify the anatomic relation with PSN, Rectal branches od IHP and HN from IHP. RVL-V (vaginal part of rectovaginal ligament)

• PSN(pelvic splanchnic nerves)

• V(vesical branches of IHP)

Inferior hypogastric plexus (IHP) and deep HN (yellow vessel loop), REC-rectal branches of inferior hypogastric plexus (IHP) (blue vessel loop)

Chapter 1

POSTOP VIEW, RIGHT

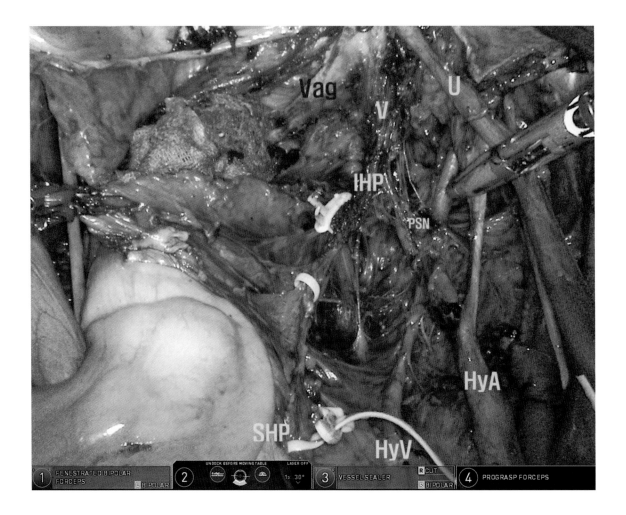

Fig. 96

This slide showed post operative view. right There were communicated with each others such as SHP(long yellow vessel loop), HN from IHP(short yellow vessel loop), rectal branches of IHP(blue vessel loop), vesical branches of IHP(V) and PSN Rectal branches of inferior hypogastric plexus(IHP) (blue vessel loop)

- HyV (hypogastric vein)
- HyA (hypogastric artery)

POSTOP VIEW, LEFT

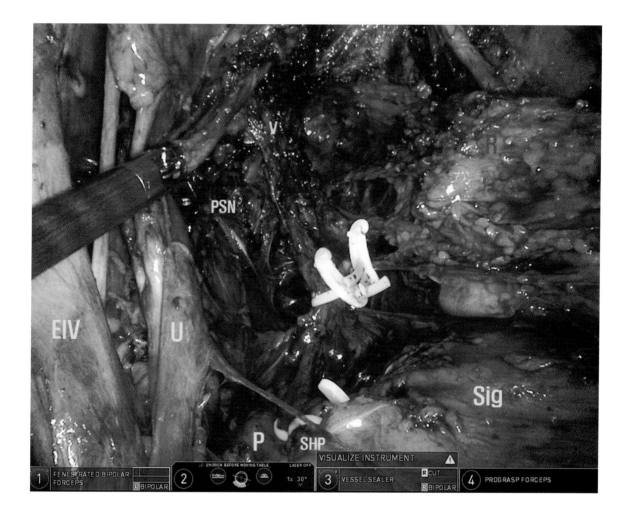

Fig. 97

This slide showed post operative view. left There were communicated with each others such as SHP(long yellow vessel loop), HN from IHP(short yellow vessel loop), rectal branches of IHP(blue vessel loop), vesical branches of IHP(V) and PSN REC-rectal branches of inferior hypogastric plexus (IHP) (blue vessel loop)

- HyV(hypogastric vein)
- HyA(hypogastric artery)
- P(promontory)

- PSN (pelvic splanchnic nerves)
- V(vesical branches of IHP)

Inferior hypogastric plexus(IHP) and deep HN(yellow vessel loop), REC-rectal branches of inferior hypogastric plexus(IHP) (blue vessel loop)

Chapter 2

Clinical outcome of Robot Extended
Nerve Sparing Radical
Hysterectomy with Extended Pelvic
Lymphadenectomy for the Cervical Cancer

Extended Nerve sparing RH
1. to preserve the rectal branches and vesical branches of inferior hypogastric plexus, so to improve the defecation and voiding function
2. to resect rectovaginal ligament for prevention of local recurrence.

Extended Pelvic Lymphadenectomy
1. to prevent isolated pelvic node recurrence

Chapter 2

CASE A ; RECURRENCE AT RECTOVAGINAL LIGAMENT

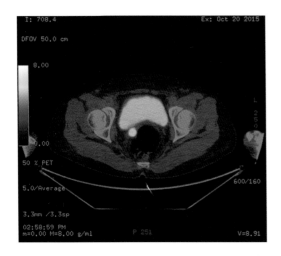

Fig. 98

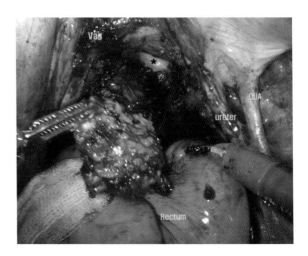

Fig. 99

Fig. 99

Case A; IB1. cervical adenocarcinoma, 49years, 2cm cancer mass, stromal invasion 62%. no node metastasis(0/42), Lymphovascular invasion +, parametrial invasion, but lower uterine segment invasion +, 9month later after single port laparoscopic radical hysterectomy, she had recurrence at vaginal part of right rectovaginal ligament..

Fig 100

This slide showed robot assisted metastatectomy. metastatic mass was located at vaginal part of rectovaginal ligament. And recur mass was far from the ureter. After operation, she had CCRT and alive without disease at 2.6 years after treatment.

Black * indicated pelvic floor muscle.

CASE B ; RECURRENCE AT RECTOVAGINAL LIGAMENT

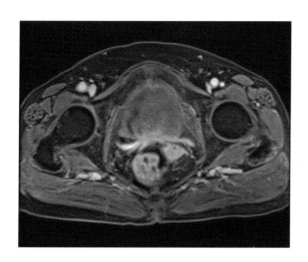

Fig. 100

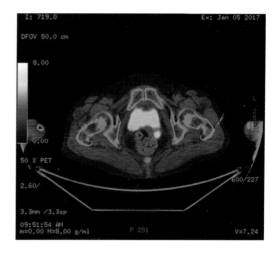

Fig. 100-1

Case B ; 73 years stage IIIA neoadjuvant chemotherapy, lymphovascular invasion, Parametrial Invasion, 72% stromal invasion, SCC, vaginal invasion+, vaginal margin clear.13 month later she had recurrence at left vaginal part of rectovaginal ligament after she had CCRT, she had complete response (Fig.101 MRI, Fig. 101-1 PET CT)

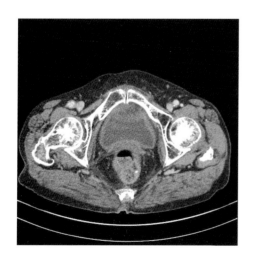

Fig. 101

This slide (pelvic CT) showed the complete response at 4months after CCRT

Chapter 2

CASE C ;
LYMPHATIC INVASION AT RECTOVAGINAL LIGAMENT

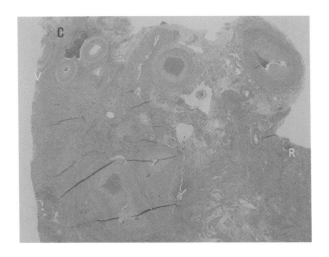

Fig. 102

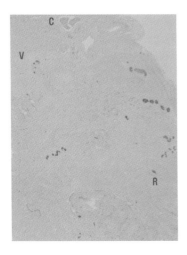

Fig. 103

Case C; 43 years, stage Ib1 SCC cervical cancer The pathologic report of right rectovaginal ligament revealed lymphatic invasion of SCC.

- V: vaginal side of RVL
- R: rectal side of RVL
- C: lymphatic metastasis

This pathologic evidence revealed that rectovaginal ligament was import ant spreading pathway of local direct spread.

Fig. 103

immunostaining of rectovaginal ligament with S-100. But there were several neural part at rectal side of rectovaginal ligament after selective preservation of rectal branches of inferior hypogastric plexus.

Conclusion ;

We proposed that the local direct spread of cervical cancer was to the uterosacral, rectovaginal (rectouterine) ligament. Which was shown by pathologic slides and recurrent cases of cervical cancer. And during the isolation of hypogastric nerve from inferior hypogastric plexus or rectal branches of Inferior hypogastric plexus, neural plane was thick, firm , elastic so it was difficult to perforate, it was need more forces to perforate. Therefore these neural plane might be barrier to direct cancer spread to lateral pelvic sidewall. Therefore, We should pay attention to resect the rectovaginal ligament.

CLINICAL OUTCOMES

2015 Mar to 2017 June, we had 53 cases of robot extended nerve sparing radical hysterectomy with extended pelvic lymphadenectomy for cervical cancer

Table 1. perioperative outcomes

Age	Mean± SD (range)
	50.6± 11.3 (31- 82)
Q index	23± 3.8 (15– 30)
Op times (min)	243.7 ± 46.4 (142– 329)
Blood loss (ml)	76.1± 244.4 (15-1500)
Hospital stay(days)	9.7± 3.8 (7-30)
Perioperative complication	
Ileus	1
transfusion	3
Voiding dysfunction	1
Ureter stricture	3
Infected lymphocyst	1

Chapter 2

CLINICAL OUTCOMES

Table 2. pathologic findings.

Stage	
IA2	3
IB1	32
IB2	6
IIA	3
IIB	9 (*, **)
pathology	
Squamous cell ca	39
Adenocarcinoma	12
Adenosquamous cell ca	1
Small cell ca	1
Positive pelvic node	7 (13%)
Positive paraaortic and pelvic node Number of positive node	2 (4%)
1	3
<5	2
=> 5	4 (*)
Parametrial invasion	
Unilateral	6
Bilateral	7 (**)
Positive node & PI+	9
Negative node & PI+	4 (**)

(*)—-one patient had recurred and dead

(**)- one patient had recurred and alive with disease

CLINICAL OUTCOMES

Table 3. postoperative treatment .

Stage	Cases	High risk cases	Postoperative treatment	
IA2	3	1	1	CCRT
IB1	32	4	2	CCRT
			2	Postop. chemotherapy
IB2	6	5	2	CCRT
			3	Postop. chemotherapy
IIA	3	1	1	Postop chemotherapy
IIB	9	9	3	CCRT (*)
			6	Postop. chemotherapy(**)
	53	20 (38%)		

(*)—- one patient had recurred and dead

(**)- one patient had recurred and alive with disease

 Mean FU period 15month (3– 30 month)

Chapter 3

video

Chapter 3

1. Film for Robot extended nerve sparing radical hysterectomy with extended pelvic lymphadenectomy for the cervical cancer-For reducing local recurrence

2. Film for Robot assisted posterior dissection (resection of rectovaginal ligament) for the cervical Cancer

3. Film for robot assisted extended pelvic lymphadenectomy

4. Film for Robot radical hysterectomy with pelvic lymphadenectomy by use of vessel sealer

• You Tube

1
2
3
4

• Naver

1
2
3
4

Chapter 4

References

Chapter 4

Robot-assisted total preservation of the pelvic autonomic nerve with extended systematic lymphadenectomy as part of nerve-sparing radical hysterectomy for cervical cancer.
Lee YS, Chong GO, Lee YH, Hong DG, Cho YL, Park IS. Int J Gynecol Cancer. 2013 Jul;23(6):1133-8.
Robot versus laparoscopic nerve-sparing radical hysterectomy for cervical cancer: a comparison of the intraoperative and perioperative results of a single surgeon's initial experience.
Chong GO, Lee YH, Hong DG, Cho YL, Park IS, Lee YS. Int J Gynecol Cancer. 2013 Jul;23(6):1145-9.
Morphogenetic fields of embryonic development in locoregional cancer spread M. Höckel , Lancet Oncol., 16 (3) (2015), p. 51
Association between developmental steps in the organogenesis of the uterine cervix and locoregional progression of cervical cancer: a prospective clinicopathological analysis M. Höckel, B. Hentschel, L.-C. Horn Lancet Oncol., 15 (4) (2014), pp. 445-456
Resection of the embryologically defined uterovaginal (Mullerian) compartment and pelvic control in patients with cervical cancer: a prospective analysis M. Höckel, L.-C. Horn, N. Manthey, U.-D. Braumann, U. Wolf, G. Teichmann, et al. Lancet Oncol., 10 (7) (2009), pp. 683-692
(Laterally) extended endopelvic resection: surgical treatment of locally advanced and recurrent cancer of the uterine cervix and vagina based on ontogenetic anatomy M. Höckel, L.-C. Horn, J. Einenkel Gynecol. Oncol., 127 (2) (2012), pp. 297-302
Long-term experience with (laterally) extended endopelvic resection (LEER) in relapsed pelvic malignancies M. Höckel Curr. Oncol. Rep., 17 (3) (2015), p. 435
Pattern analysis of regional spread and therapeutic lymph node dissection in cervical cancer based on ontogenetic anatomy. M. Höckel, L.-C. Horn, E. Tetsch, J. Einenkel Gynecol. Oncol., 125 (1) (2012), pp. 168-174